D0875959

Auditory Perception
(PGPS-109)

Pergamon Titles of Related Interest

Caelli VISUAL PERCEPTION: Theory and Practice
Cohen SLEEP AND DREAMING: Origins, Nature and Functions

Related Journals*

PHYSIOLOGY AND BEHAVIOR
PSYCHONEUROENDOCRINOLOGY
VISION RESEARCH

*Free specimen copies available upon request.

PERGAMON GENERAL PSYCHOLOGY SERIES
EDITORS
Arnold P. Goldstein, *Syracuse University*
Leonard Krasner, *SUNY at Stony Brook*

Auditory Perception
A New Synthesis

Richard M. Warren
University of Wisconsin-Milwaukee

PERGAMON PRESS
New York   Oxford   Toronto   Sydney   Paris   Frankfurt

Pergamon Press Offices:

U.S.A.   Pergamon Press Inc., Maxwell House, Fairview Park,
                    Elmsford, New York 10523, U.S.A.

U.K.   Pergamon Press Ltd., Headington Hill Hall,
                    Oxford OX3 0BW, England

CANADA   Pergamon Press Canada Ltd., Suite 104, 150 Consumers Road,
                    Willowdale, Ontario M2J 1P9, Canada

AUSTRALIA   Pergamon Press (Aust.) Pty. Ltd., P.O. Box 544,
                    Potts Point, NSW 2011, Australia

FRANCE   Pergamon Press SARL, 24 rue des Ecoles,
                    75240 Paris, Cedex 05, France

FEDERAL REPUBLIC Pergamon Press GmbH, Hammerweg 6
OF GERMANY   6242 Kronberg/Taunus, Federal Republic of Germany

Copyright © 1982 Pergamon Press Inc.

Library of Congress Cataloging in Publication Data

Warren, Richard M.

    Auditory perception.

    (Pergamon general psychology series ; 109)
    Bibliography: p.
    Includes index.
    1. Auditory perception. 2. Speech perception.
I. Title. II. Series
QP461.W27   1982   152.1′5   81-23488
ISBN 0-08-025957-X   AACR2

Printed in the United States of America

To Roslyn

Contents

CHAPTER 3 PERCEPTION OF ACOUSTIC REPETITION: PITCH AND INFRAPITCH

Preface

During the course of my work in hearing over the last 25 years, I have become convinced that there is a greater interconnection between topics in auditory perception than is generally appreciated. This book attempts to show interrelations between major areas in hearing. Each chapter reviews the history of classical problems as well as current evidence and interpretations, with emphasis on work from my laboratory when applicable.

While it is hoped that this book will be of value to research scientists and to professionals working in speech and hearing, no detailed specialized knowledge is assumed. Basic information necessary for understanding the material covered is provided, so that it may be used in courses for advanced undergraduate and graduate students in behavioral sciences, neurobiology, engineering, and the health sciences and professions.

My research described here was carried out at the following institutions: Brown University; New York University College of Medicine; Cambridge University; Oxford University; The Medical Research Council Applied Psychology Unit, Cambridge, England; The Laboratory of Psychology at The National Institute of Mental Health; and The University of Wisconsin-Milwaukee. I am grateful for extramural support from the National Institutes of Health and from the National Science Foundation over the years, as well as a Senior Postdoctoral Fellowship in Physiological Psychology from the National Research Council of the National Academy of Sciences, and for support from the University of Wisconsin-Milwaukee.

I wish to thank Susan E. Galloway for her dedicated work in typing and retyping, as well as Ellen K. Throgmorton and Joan M. Zarzynski for helping her with this task. I am grateful to Marilyn Budhal and Laurie Fike for their work on the figures.

I acknowledge my debt to my graduate students past and present, especially to John M. Ackroff, James A. Bashford, Jr., Brad S. Brubaker,

Charles J. Obusek, Julian L. Puretz, Gary L. Sherman, and John M. Wrightson.

I am very grateful to Ivan Hunter-Duvar at the Hospital for Sick Children, Toronto, for providing the excellent scanning electron micrograph appearing as figure 1.8, and to Alvin M. Liberman of Haskins Laboratory, New Haven, Connecticut, for providing the original photograph used for figure 7.6.

I am especially indebted to Robert A. Butler, Joseph E. Hind, and Reinier Plomp for their valuable suggestions and comments concerning an earlier draft. David S. Emmerich's editorial comments have been invaluable.

Finally, I acknowledge the essential role of Roslyn Pauker Warren, my colleague and wife. Without her, this book would not have been started, and once started could not have been finished.

Auditory Perception
(PGPS-109)

1

Sound and
the Auditory System

This chapter provides a brief introduction to the physical nature of sound, the manner in which it is transmitted and transformed within the ear, and the nature of auditory neural responses.

THE NATURE OF AUDITORY STIMULI

Understanding hearing requires an understanding of sound. Sounds consist of fluctuations in pressure which are propagated through an elastic medium, and are associated with displacement of particles composing the medium. When the substance conducting sound is air at a temperature and pressure within the normal environmental ranges, compressions and rarefactions are transmitted at a velocity of about 335 meters per second, regardless of their amplitude (extent of pressure change) or waveform (pattern of pressure changes over time). Special interest is attached to periodic sounds, or sounds having a fixed waveform repeated at a fixed frequency. Frequency is measured in Hertz (Hz) or numbers of repetitions of a waveform per second (thus, 1,000 Hz corresponds to 1,000 repetitions of a particular waveform per second). The time required for one complete statement of an iterated waveform is its period. Periodic sounds from about 20 through 16,000 Hz can produce a sensation of pitch, and are called tones. For reasons to be discussed shortly, it is generally considered that the simplest type of periodic sound is a sine wave or pure tone (shown in Fig. 1.1A) which has a sinusoidal change in pressure over time. A limitless number of other periodic waveforms exist, including square waves (Fig. 1.1B) and pulse trains (Fig. 1.1C). Periodic sounds need not have simple, symmetrical waveforms: figure 1.1D shows a periodic sound produced by iteration of a randomly generated waveform.

1

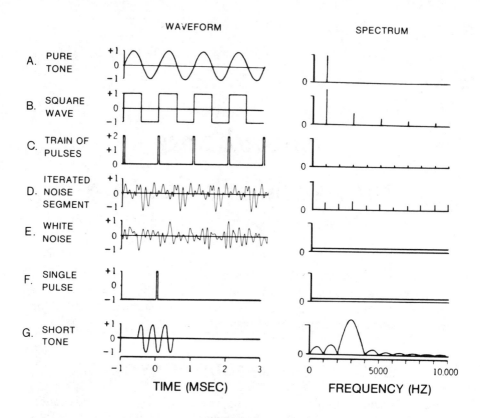

Fig. 1.1. Waveforms and amplitude spectra. The periodic waveforms have line spectra, and the nonperiodic waveforms have continuous spectra or band spectra. See text for further discussion.

The figure also depicts the waveforms of some nonperiodic sounds: white or Gaussian noise (Fig. 1.1E), a single pulse (Fig. 1.1F), and a short tone or tone burst (Fig. 1.1G).

    The waveforms shown in figure 1.1 are time-domain representations in which both amplitude and time are depicted. Using a procedure developed by Joseph Fourier in the first half of the nineteenth century, it also is possible to represent any periodic sound in terms of a frequency-domain or spectral analysis in which a sound is described in terms of a harmonic sequence of sinusoidal components having appropriate frequency, amplitude, and phase relations. (Phase describes the portion of the period through which a wave-form has advanced relative to an arbitrary reference.) A sinusoidal tone

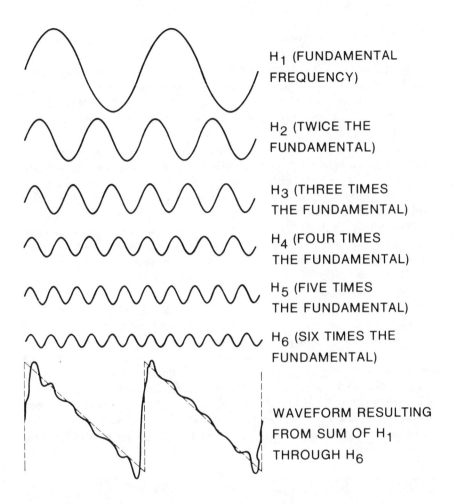

H_1 (FUNDAMENTAL FREQUENCY)

H_2 (TWICE THE FUNDAMENTAL)

H_3 (THREE TIMES THE FUNDAMENTAL)

H_4 (FOUR TIMES THE FUNDAMENTAL)

H_5 (FIVE TIMES THE FUNDAMENTAL)

H_6 (SIX TIMES THE FUNDAMENTAL)

WAVEFORM RESULTING FROM SUM OF H_1 THROUGH H_6

Fig. 1.2. Synthesis of a complex waveform through addition of harmonically related sinusoidal components. The approximation of a sawtooth waveform could be made closer by the addition of higher harmonics of appropriate amplitude and phase.

Source: From Perception and the Senses by Evan L. Brown and Kenneth Deffenbacher. Copyright 1979 by Oxford University Press, Inc. Reprinted by permission.

consists of a single spectral component as shown in figure 1.1A. The figure also shows the power spectra corresponding to the particular complex (nonsinusoidal) periodic sounds shown in figures 1.1B, 1.1C, and 1.1D. Each of these sounds has a period of 1 millisecond, a fundamental frequency of 1,000 Hz (corresponding to the waveform repetition frequency), and harmonic components corresponding to integral multiples of the 1,000 Hz fundamental as indicated.

Frequency analysis is not restricted to periodic sounds: nonperiodic sounds also have a spectral composition as defined through use of a Fourier integral or Fourier transform (for details see Leshowitz, 1978). Nonperiodic sounds have continuous rather than line spectra, as shown for the sounds depicted in figures 1.1E, 1.1F, and 1.1G.

As we shall see, frequency analysis of both periodic and nonperiodic sounds is of particular importance in hearing, chiefly because the ear performs a crude spectral analysis before the auditory receptors are stimulated.

While figure 1.1 shows how particular waveforms can be analyzed in terms of spectral components, it is also possible to synthesize waveforms by adding together sinusoidal components of appropriate phase and amplitude. Figure 1.2 shows how a sawtooth waveform may be approximated closely by the mixing of only six harmonics having appropriate amplitude and phase.

The range of audible amplitude changes is very large. A sound producing discomfort may be as much as 10^6 times the amplitude level at threshold. Sound level can be measured as power or intensity as well as amplitude or pressure: power usually can be considered as proportional to the square of the amplitude, so that discomfort occurs at a power level 10^{12} times the power threshold. In order to span the large range of values needed to describe the levels of sound normally encountered, a logarithmic scale has been devised. The logarithm to the base 10 of the ratio of a particular sound power level to a reference power level defines the level of the sound in Bels (named in honor of Alexander Graham Bell). However, the Bel is a rather large unit, and it is conventional to use a unit 1/10 this size, the deciBel (or dB) to express sound levels. The level in dB can be defined as:

$$dB = 10 \log_{10} I_1/I_2$$

where I_1 is the power level of the particular sound of interest, and I_2 is the reference level expressed as sound power. DeciBels can also be calculated on the basis of amplitude or pressure units using the equation:

$$dB = 20 \log_{10} P_1/P_2$$

where P_1 is the relative pressure level being measured, and P_2 is the reference pressure level. The standard reference pressure level is 0.0002 dyne/cm^2 (which is sometimes expressed in different units of 20 microPascals), and the level in dB measured relative to this standard is called Sound Pressure Level (or SPL). Sound level meters are calibrated so that the numerical value of the SPL can be read out directly. There is another measure of sound level, also expressed in dB, called Sensation Level (SL), which is used occasionally in psychoacoustics. When measuring SL, the intensity corresponding to the threshold of a sound for an individual listener is used as the reference level rather than the standard physical value employed for SPL, so that dB SL represents the level above an individual's threshold. Since SL is used relatively infrequently, dB will always refer to SPL unless otherwise specified.

To give some feeling for intensity levels in dB, the threshold of normal listeners for a 1,000 Hz sinusoidal tone is about 6 dB, the ambient level (background noise) in radio and TV studios is about 30 dB, conversational speech about 55 dB, and the level inside a bus about 90 dB.

Experimenters can vary the relative intensities of spectral components by use of acoustic filters which, in analogy with light filters, pass only desired frequency components of a sound. A high-pass filter transmits only frequency components above a lower limit, a low-pass filter only frequencies below an upper limit. Band-pass filters (which transmit frequencies within a specified range) and band-reject filters (which block frequencies within a specified range) are available. Filters are specified in terms of both cut-off frequency (the frequency at which the filter attenuation reaches 3 dB), and the slope, or roll-off, which is usually expressed as dB/octave beyond the cut-off frequency (an increase of one octave corresponds to doubling the frequency). Filter types are shown in figure 1.3.

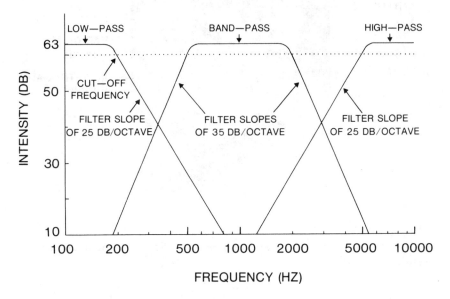

Fig. 1.3. Characteristics of filters. Low-pass, high-pass, and band-pass filters are shown, with filter slopes (dB/octave) and cut-off frequencies (frequencies at which there is a 3 dB reduction in intensity) illustrated.

OUR AUDITORY APPARATUS

The Outer Ear and the Middle Ear

It is convenient to consider the ear as consisting of three divisions. The outer ear (also called the pinna or auricle) is shown in figure 1.4. It appears to contribute to localization of sound sources by virtue of its direction-specific effect on the intensity of certain frequency components of sounds, as will be discussed in a later chapter. The human pinna is surrounded by a simple flange (the helix) which is extended considerably in some other mammals to form a conical structure functioning as a short version of the old-fashioned ear trum-

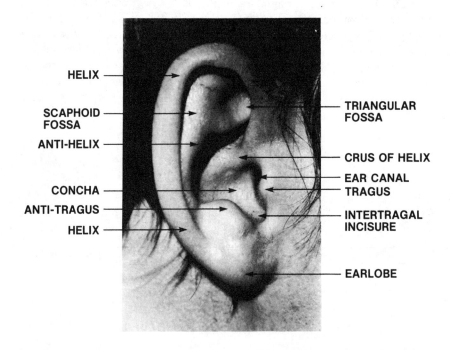

HELIX

SCAPHOID FOSSA

ANTI-HELIX

CONCHA

ANTI-TRAGUS

HELIX

TRIANGULAR FOSSA

CRUS OF HELIX

EAR CANAL

TRAGUS

INTERTRAGAL INCISURE

EARLOBE

Fig. 1.4. The outer ear (other names: pinna and auricle). The major anatomical features are shown.

pet. These ear-cones increase the sensitivity of such animals to high frequency sounds when pointed toward their source by controlling muscles, as well as providing information concerning azimuth of the source.

After the acoustic transformation produced by reflections within our pinna, the sound passes through the ear canal (or external auditory meatus) which ends at the eardrum or tympanum as shown in figure 1.5. This canal is more than a passive conduit. Its length is roughly 2.5 cm, and it behaves in some respects like a resonant tube, such as an organ pipe. The effect of this resonance is to amplify frequencies appreciably (5 dB or more) from about 2,000 through 5,500 Hz, with a maximum amplification of about 11 dB occurring at about 4,000 Hz (Wiener, 1947). The pressure changes at the end of the canal cause the tympanum to vibrate. This vibration is picked up and transmitted by a chain of three small bones or ossicles located in the middle ear. The first of these bones, the malleus (or hammer) is attached to the tympanum, and its movement is transmitted to the incus (or anvil) and thence to

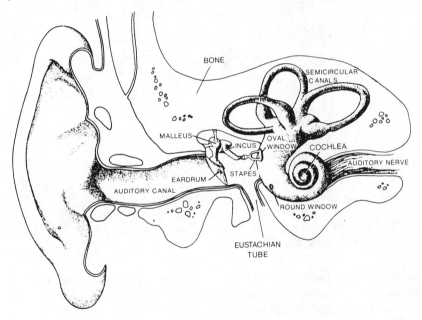

Fig. 1.5. Diagram of the entire ear. The outer, middle, and inner ear are shown, along with adjacent structures.
Source: Adapted from P.H. Lindsay and D.A. Norman, *Human Information Processing: An Introduction to Psychology.* (2nd ed.) (New York: Academic Press, 1977).

the stapes (or stirrup). The stapes is connected to the oval window at the base of the fluid-filled cochlea. This window lies at the boundary of the middle and inner ears. The passage of sound through the cochlea is shown in figure 1.6, and will be discussed subsequently.

The middle ear permits the air-borne sound to be converted to liquid-borne sound without the great loss which would otherwise occur. When sound in air impinges directly upon a liquid, a loss of about 30 dB (99.9 percent of the power) takes place, with most of the sound energy being reflected back into the air. Three physical principles act to increase the efficiency of the transmission of sound by the middle ear: (1) the curvature of the tympanum

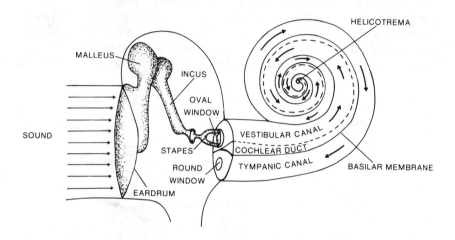

Fig. 1.6. Conversion from air-borne to liquid-borne motion by the ear.
Source: Adapted from P.H. Lindsay and D.A. Norman, *Human Information Processing: An Introduction to Psychology* (2nd ed.) (New York: Academic Press, 1977).

(which is somewhat conical in shape) causes it to act like a more efficient mechanical transformer (Tonndorf & Khanna, 1972); (2) the chain of three ossicles acts like a lever with a small mechanical advantage; and (3) the force applied to the larger area of the tympanic membrane, when transmitted to the much smaller area of the footplate of the stapes embedded in the oval window, produces a considerable mechanical advantage. (This last factor is the most important of the three.)

There are two muscles within the middle ear which can lessen the intensity of very strong stimuli and minimize the possibility of damage to the inner ear. One of these (the tensor tympani muscle) is attached to the malleus, and the other (the stapedius muscle) is attached to the stapes. These muscles are sometimes compared in their effect to the iris of the eye—a high level of stimulus intensity causes a reflex contraction of the muscles resulting in a decrease in stimulation. Once the threshold for initiating the reflex is reached, there is a maximum decrease in intensity of about 0.6 or 0.7 dB for each dB above this threshold, with an upper limit of perhaps 30 dB for low frequency sounds (the reduction in intensity is greatest for low frequency components). Middle ear muscle contraction also can reduce distortions which would otherwise occur from overloading the ossicular chain. Very few people can contract their middle ear muscles voluntarily. For most of us the action is strictly reflexive, either in response to an external sound of 80 dB or more, or as an action which precedes the self-generation of sound in speaking or chewing of food. The reflex activity of these muscles in response to external sound is very quick, perhaps 10 msec for very intense sounds, but this still cannot protect against sudden harmful sounds such as gunshots.

Are the intra-aural muscles more than an analog of the eye's iris? There are some interesting speculations. Lawrence (1965) suggested that, since animal studies have indicated that muscle activity is to some degree independent in the two ears, intermittent monaural changes in intensity and phase produced by muscle contraction can help in directing attention to sources at different azimuths under noisy conditions. Simmons (1964) considered that low frequency sounds produced by chewing and by head movements might mask high frequency environmental sounds of importance, and selective attenuation of these self-generated sounds by coordinated reflex contraction of the intra-aural muscles could permit detection of such external sounds.

Structure of the Inner Ear

The inner ear contains not only the organ of hearing, but also organs involved in detecting acceleration and maintaining balance. The complex structure of the inner ear has led to its being called the labyrinth. The vestibule of the labyrinth contains the utricle and saccule which appear to be sensitive to linear acceleration of the head and to orientation in the gravitational field. There are also three bony semicircular canals, each set at right angles to the other two, which can detect rotary acceleration in any plane (see Fig. 1.5). The bony spiral structure within the inner ear called the cochlea (from the Latin name for snail) contains the organ for hearing. This coiled tube consists of about 2.5 turns and has a length of about 3.5 cm. It is partitioned into three canals or ducts called scalae. Two of the scalae are joined: the scala vestibuli or vestibular canal (which has at its basal end the flexible oval window to which the stapes is attached) communicates (via a small opening called the helicotrema at the apex of the spiral) with the scala tympani or tympanic canal (which has the flexible round window at its basal end). These two scalae contain a fluid called perilymph, and when the oval window is flexed inward by the stapes, the almost incompressible perilymph causes the round window to flex outward. As shown in figure 1.7, the scala vestibuli is bounded by Reissner's membrane and the scala tympani by the basilar membrane. Between these two membranes lies the scala media or cochlear duct, which has a closed end near the helicotrema and which contains a fluid called endolymph. A third fluid called cortilymph is found within the tunnel of Corti.

Auditory receptors are found within a complex neuroepithelium called the organ of Corti lying on the basilar membrane. The receptors are of two types: the outer hair cells (which are closer to the cochlear wall) found in three rows, and a single row of inner hair cells. Each hair cell is topped by a plate containing stereocilia. The stereocilia are bathed in endolymph, while

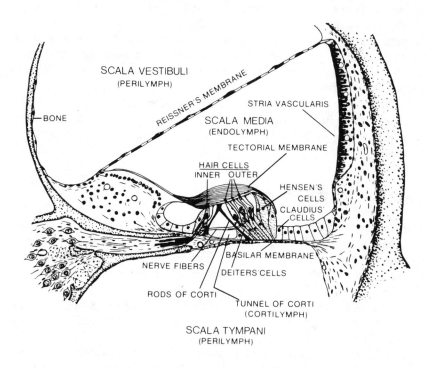

Fig. 1.7. Cross-section of the cochlea, showing the organ of Corti and associated structures. This diagram is based on the guinea pig, but is representative of the human inner ear as well.

Source: Adapted from H. Davis, R.W. Benson, W.P. Covell, C. Fernandez, R. Goldstein, Y. Katsuki, J.P. Legouix, D.R. McAuliffe, and I. Tasaki, "Acoustic Trauma in the Guinea Pig," *Journal of the Acoustical Society of America* 25 (1953): 1180-89.

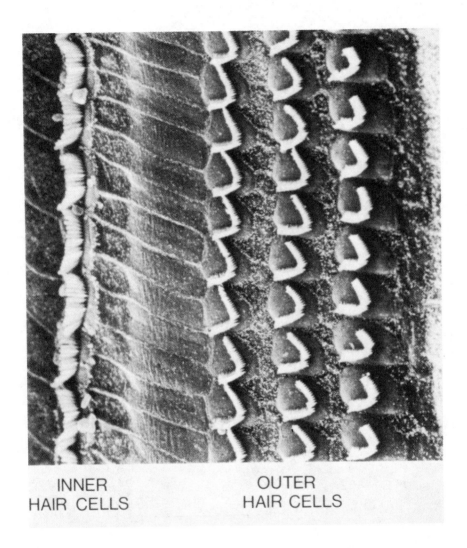

INNER
HAIR CELLS

OUTER
HAIR CELLS

Fig. 1.8. Scanning electron micrograph of the top of the organ of Corti. The tectorial membrane has been removed to expose the stereocilia and upper surfaces of the outer hair cells (three rows) and the inner hair cells (one row). (Chinchilla photograph courtesy of Dr. Ivan Hunter-Dewar, Hospital for Sick Children, Toronto.)

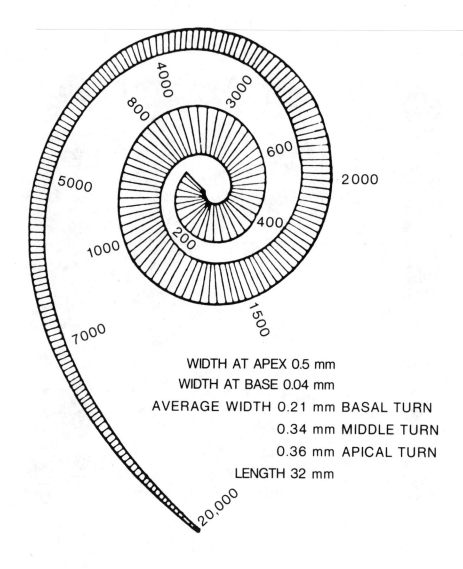

WIDTH AT APEX 0.5 mm
WIDTH AT BASE 0.04 mm
AVERAGE WIDTH 0.21 mm BASAL TURN
0.34 mm MIDDLE TURN
0.36 mm APICAL TURN
LENGTH 32 mm

Fig. 1.9. Diagram of the human basilar membrane, showing the approximate positions of maximal displacement to tones of different frequencies, and changes in width going from the base (near the stapes and oval window) to the apex (near the helicotrema). The ratio of width to length is exaggerated to show the variation in width more clearly.

Source: From O. Stuhlman, Jr., *An Introduction to Biophysics* (New York: Wiley, 1943).

most of the receptor cell is surrounded by cortilymph. Outer hair cells each contain about 100 stereocilia arranged in the form of a letter V or W; the inner hair cells each contain about 50 stereocilia generally in two roughly parallel rows (see Fig. 1.8). The tips of some stereocilia may be embedded in the tectorial membrane, the tips of others may move with the tectorial membrane because of attachment by thin fibrils, or perhaps because of viscous forces. It seems that a shearing deflection of these stereocilia causes electrochemical changes in the receptor cells leading to stimulation of the associated auditory nerve fibers.

The basilar membrane is tapered, with a width of about 0.04 mm at the base increasing to 0.5 mm at the helicotrema (see Fig. 1.9). In addition to becoming wider with increasing distance from the stapes and oval window, the basilar membrane decreases in its stiffness—the displacement to a constant force (its compliance) increases by a factor of almost 100 in going from the basal end to the apex. These features seem to result in a "tuning" to different frequencies of sound along the basilar membrane. As shown in figure 1.9, the region near the stapes shows maximum displacement amplitude to high frequencies, and the region near the helicotrema shows its greatest displacement to low frequencies. The frequency selectivity resembles a Fourier analysis of limited resolution. This is a topic of great importance to theories of hearing, and will be discussed in more detail in the section dealing with cochlear mechanics.

All of the blood reaching the cochlea comes through the internal auditory artery. Since there is no collateral source of blood, all structures within the cochlea degenerate if this blood supply is cut off. Capillaries are found below (not within) the basilar membrane and on the wall of the cochlear duct some distance from the auditory receptor cells, so that nutrients and metabolic products are transported by diffusion through the endolymph. This spatial separation of the capillaries reduces the sound associated with blood circulation at the location of the auditory receptors. Even with this increased distance from capillaries, there is still a relatively high level of low frequency noise at the receptors caused by blood circulation (which is not heard because of the high threshold of the auditory system for low frequency sounds).

Neural Structures and Auditory Pathways

Innervation of the auditory receptor cells is by the auditory nerve, which is also known as the cochlear branch of the vestibulocochlear (VIIIth) nerve. There are about 30,000 auditory nerve fibers associated with each inner ear. Their peripheral terminations consist of dendritic endings surrounding the inner and the outer hair cells, and their central terminations are associated with neurons in the dorsal and ventral cochlear nuclei located within the lower brainstem (the medulla oblongata).

The nerve fibers lose their myelin sheaths before entering the organ of Corti. They enter through openings near the inner hair cells called the habenula perforata, with about eight or nine fibers passing through each of the openings. Over 90 percent of these afferent fibers terminate on inner hair cells, with individual hair cells innervated by about eight separate fibers. The few remaining afferent fibers cross the tunnel of Corti, make a right-angle turn toward the basal end, and send out collateral branches which innervate the outer hair cells. About 10 outer cells are connected with each fiber, with each outer hair cell making contact with perhaps three or four separate fibers.

The first order afferent or ascending auditory fibers all terminate at the cochlear nucleus. A number of different routes are available within the ascending pathway leading to the cortex. Some of the brainstem nuclei and their interconnections are shown in figure 1.10. The ventral part of the cochlear nucleus sends second order fibers to both the ipsilateral and the contralateral superior olive and the accessory superior olive. The dorsal cochlear nucleus sends second order axons to the contralateral lateral lemniscus and inferior colliculus. Some third order neurons also reach the inferior colliculus after synapsing with second order neurons in the dorsal nucleus of the lateral lemniscus. In addition, the inferior colliculus receives fibers from the contralateral accessory nucleus of the superior olive and the ipsilateral superior olive and accessory olive. From the colliculus, fibers go to both the reticular formation and to the medial geniculate. There are no connections between the two medial geniculates so that all subcortical lateral interactions occur below this level. The auditory cortex is located within the temporal lobes. There is a lateral asymmetry in auditory cortical processing: the left hemisphere plays a dominant role in speech perception for most people, and other types of auditory processing also show evidence of dominance of one hemisphere or the other (Kimura, 1967). While information reaching one cochlea is transmitted to both hemispheres, under some conditions contralateral transmission seems favored over ipsilateral. (For a review of this literature, see Berlin & McNeil, 1976.) However, there is a richly innervated connection between hemispheres via the corpus callosum.

There are four or five synapses along the route from cochlea to cortex, with an increase of complexity of interconnections as we ascend the auditory pathway. In humans, the 30,000 fibers within each of the two auditory nerves feed into the roughly 1 million subcortical neurons on each side associated with the auditory pathway to the cortex. The cochlear nucleus has about 90,000 neurons, the superior olivary complex (together with the trapezoid body) 34,000, the lateral lemniscus 38,000, the inferior colliculus 400,000, the medial geniculate 500,000, and the auditory cortex 100 million (Worden, 1971).

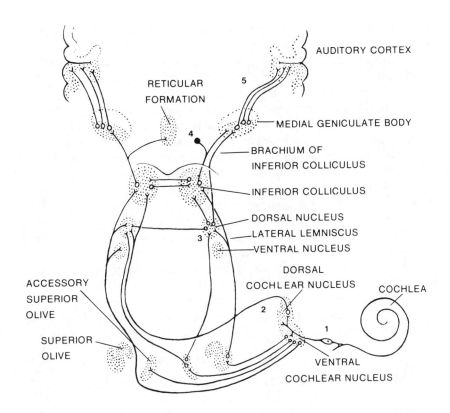

Fig. 1.10. Major structures in the ascending (afferent) chain from cochlea to cortex and some of the interconnections between structures. The numbers indicate the neuron levels (or orders).
Source: From R.R. Gacek, "Neuroanatomy of the Auditory System," in J.V. Tobias (Ed.), *Foundations of Modern Auditory Theory*. Vol. 2 (New York: Academic Press, 1972), pp. 241-62.

While the nature of interactions and processing of information along the afferent auditory pathway is obscure, the large number of neurons within subcortical centers relative to the number of auditory nerve fibers indicates the importance of subcortical processing. Hence, the conventional term of auditory "pathway" can be misleading, since it implies a passive conduit from receptor cells to cortex.

In addition to the afferent or ascending fibers carrying information from the organ of Corti, there are also efferent or descending fibers carrying impulses from higher centers down to their terminations on the inner and outer hair cells. The fibers form the olivocochlear bundle in the cochlear nerve with cell bodies located in the superior olivary regions. Some of the cell bodies are ipsilateral and some are contralateral relative to the cochlea at which their fibers terminate. While the olivocochlear bundle was originally described by Rasmussen (1946, 1953) for animals other than man, this efferent bundle has been reported for man as well (Gacek, 1961). Extrapolation from Rasmussen's detailed observation on the cat indicates that, while there may be only several hundred efferent fibers entering the cochlea, very extensive ramifications result in tens of thousands of terminations on hair cells, with the great majority associated directly with outer hair cells. For the few efferents associated with the inner hair cells, it appears that contact generally is made through synapses with dendrites of afferent fibers, with only a small proportion of connections made directly with inner hair cells. Experiments in which the olivocochlear bundle was cut generally have indicated that, while thresholds remain unchanged for tones, there may be some loss of the ability to discriminate between frequencies attributable to the loss of efferent function.

In addition to containing cell bodies of the efferent auditory system, the superior olivary complex is involved in both the reflex contraction of the middle ear muscles and the eyeblink reflex accompanying sudden loud sounds.

Mechanics for Stimulation within the Inner Ear

The mechanical responses within the inner ear leading to stimulation of the auditory receptor cells are quite complex. In the nineteenth century, Helmholtz suggested that the inner ear performs a frequency (or Fourier) analysis of sounds, with different regions of the organ of Corti vibrating maximally to different frequency components. He considered that the spectrum was spread out along the basilar membrane, starting with the highest frequencies at the basal end, and the lowest frequencies at the apical end. The location of the stimulated nerve fibers, according to Helmholtz, signaled the frequency components of the sounds. His initial theory (presented in the first edition of his *Sensations of Tone* in 1863) suggested that the rods of Corti located near the nerve fibers on the basilar membrane (see Fig. 1.7) might furnish resonators for the spectral components by virtue of gradations in stiffness and tension. Subsequent studies indicated that the rods of Corti were absent in birds and amphibia; and this, together with new evidence showing that there was a graded increase in width of the basilar membrane in the direction of the apex (see Fig. 1.9), caused Helmholtz to change his suggestion concerning the resonating elements. His second suggestion was that the basilar membrane itself was set into sympathetic vibration due to appropriately stretched and loaded radial fibers located within the membrane. These fibers, so the

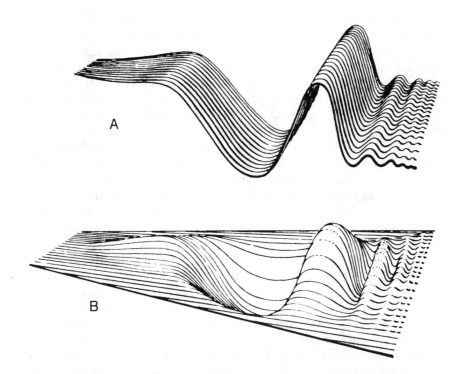

Fig. 1.11. Two models of the traveling wave pattern along the basilar membrane: (A) represents the momentary displacement of a ribbon-like model; (B) represents a refinement of (A) in which displacement is shown for a ribbon attached at both edges.
Source: From J. Tonndorf, "Shearing Motion in Scala Media of Cochlear Models," *Journal of the Acoustical Society of America* 32 (1960): 238-44.

theory went, provided high frequency resonance at the basal end and low frequency resonance at the apical end (see Helmholtz, 1954, for translation conformal with the 4th German edition, 1877). This second version of his place theory is the one generally remembered today, although we shall return later to his first theory involving the rods of Corti. In his revised place theory, Helmholtz did not propose that the resonance of a fiber within the basilar membrane was limited to a narrow range of frequencies, but that appreciable vibration of the fiber would still occur when the frequency was removed as much as a semitone from that producing maximal response.

Békésy, in a series of experiments having great impact on theories of cochlear mechanics (for summary see Békésy, 1960), claimed that, while movement of the basilar membrane provided a basis for frequency analysis involving place of stimulation, the details were rather different than those envisioned by Helmholtz. Békésy examined preparations of the basilar membrane through a microscope and observed that fine glass filaments with rounded tips pressed against the membrane produced a circular deformation, rather than the elliptical pattern which would be predicted from the transverse tension postulated by Helmholtz. (However, Voldrich, 1978, has questioned the validity of Békésy's observations.) Békésy also claimed that, when the basilar membrane was cut, the edges did not gape apart in a lens-shaped opening, as should occur were there lateral tension. Rather, the edges of the cut did not draw apart at all, indicating that there was little tension in any direction. Békésy likened the basilar membrane to a gelatinous sheet, and suggested that graded differences in the width and the stiffness of the basilar membrane are responsible for differences in the locus of maximal displacement by traveling waves. Perhaps the simplest type of traveling wave to visualize is one which sweeps down a rope attached to a fixed support at one end when it is given a shake at the other. However, a traveling wave on the basilar membrane has some features not found in this very simple model. The velocity of the traveling wave on the basilar membrane is not constant, changing from 105 m/sec when 20 mm from the oval window, to about 10 m/sec near the apex. The speed of sound in the cochlear liquids is very much faster, about 1,600 m/sec. Thus, the traveling wave occurs later than the compression wave corresponding to sound transmission in the cochlear fluids. The traveling wave (see Fig. 1.11) always moves in the direction from basal to apical end regardless of the direction of the compression wave. Even when the compression wave is made to travel in an antidromic direction from apex to base, the traveling wave still originates at the base and travels in the usual fashion toward the apex. The hydrodynamic principles governing production of the traveling wave through the exchange of energy between the basilar membrane and the surrounding fluids are discussed in detail by Dallos (1978). The physical principles involved in the production of the traveling wave interact in an extremely complex fashion, making an exact analytic solution impossible. However, approximate solutions become possible using several simplifying assumptions.

Since the maximal displacement of the basilar membrane occurs at different loci for different frequencies (as shown in Fig. 1.9), the membrane functions as a filter producing a spectral analysis of sound. The basal end responds maximally to high frequencies, and these spectral elements are removed as components of the traveling wave as it continues its passage along the basilar membrane. The lower frequency components are present at loci responding maximally to higher frequencies, although these lower frequencies produce motions of relatively small magnitude at these positions. The first direct observations of such motions were made by Békésy who used an optical microscope to view cochleae obtained from cadavers. He also viewed motions produced by traveling waves along the basilar membrane using a series of mammals ranging in size from a mouse to an elephant. Detection of motion using an optical microscope is limited to resolution of displacements of 1 micrometer or more, corresponding to very high sound intensities (120 dB and above). Also, Békésy's detailed observations were limited to the more accessible apical half of the basilar membrane. After his pioneering studies, more sensitive methods for measuring basilar membrane motion became available. One is the Mössbauer technique first employed in the study of cochlear mechanics by Johnstone and Boyle (1967) and Johnstone, Taylor, and Boyle (1970). In this procedure, a tiny bit of radioactive substance (a gamma ray emitter) is placed on the basilar membrane, the added mass being considered small enough not to interfere appreciably with vibratory movement. The Doppler effect produced by motion of the gamma ray source toward and away from the detector causes small frequency shifts. Usually Cobalt-57 atoms locked into a crystalline lattice are used as the radioactive source: decay produces excited Iron-57 atoms, which remain in the same lattice position (minimizing inertial recoil) when emitting a gamma ray of characteristic fixed frequency to become stable Iron-57. A screen of stable (nonexcited) Iron-57 placed between emitter and detector serves as a very sharply tuned filter which absorbs the gamma rays when the emitter lying upon the basilar membrane is at rest. Vibration of the basilar membrane results in Doppler shifts in frequency which permit the radiation to pass through the filter to a detector. This technique was also used by Rhode (1971, 1973) to show that the mechanical properties of the basilar membrane are quite different in live and dead animals, with changes appearing quite rapidly after death. Kohllöffel (1972a, 1972b, 1972c) used laser illumination of the basilar membrane to determine incoherence or "speckling" of reflected images caused by the Doppler effect with both live and dead guinea pigs, obtaining results in general agreement with those found with the Mössbauer method. In addition, Wilson and Johnstone (1975) used a very sensitive capacitance probe to measure the mechanical filter characteristics of the basilar membrane.

Each of the methods used to measure the filter characteristics of the basilar membrane indicates that frequency resolution is not as sharp as that observed by measuring the electrophysiological responses of nerve fibers or psychophysical (behavioral) responses. This has led to the suggestion that sharpening may occur through lateral inhibition(or lateral suppression)produced in regions surrounding those of maximal stimulation (Békésy, 1960; Houtgast, 1974a), or through interactions between waves produced along the basilar membrane through longitudinal coupling with the tectorial membrane (Zwislocki, 1980; Zwislocki & Kletsky, 1979). An especially interesting hypothesis is that sharpening may involve resonant frequencies of the stereocilia—a possibility reminiscent of Helmholtz's initial resonance theory (discussed earlier) involving resonance of the rods of Corti rather than the hypothetical transverse fibers within the basilar membrane suggested in his revised theory. Flock, Flock, and Murray (1977) reported that stereocilia form stiff bundles which move as a unit. This observation, together with Lim's (1980) evidence that both inner and outer hair cells' cilia are tallest at the apex and shortest at the base of the cochlea, suggest that stereocilia may be tuned to particular frequencies, and so may sharpen the filter characteristics of the basilar membrane. It also has been suggested by Hudspeth and Jacobs (1979) that the stiffness of the stereocilia (which contain actin also found in muscle fibers) can be modulated by intracellular calcium ions (which also can modulate muscle contraction) so that tuning may be under metabolic control. Perhaps some efferent neural influence could be exerted via this metabolic route.

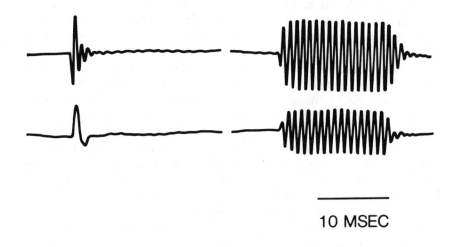

10 MSEC

Fig. 1.12. Cochlear microphonic response to a click (left) and tone burst (right) in the guinea pig. The upper tracings represent the cochlear microphonic response measured with difference electrodes, the lower tracings depict the acoustic waveforms monitored at the eardrum.
Source: From P. Dallos, *The Auditory Periphery: Biophysics and Physiology* (New York: Academic Press, 1973).

There have been reports that detectable tone-like narrow band sounds can be emitted by the ear, suggesting some active physiological process within the cochlea. In one case, this "objective tinnitus" or ringing by the ear was loud enough to be heard by people nearby (Huizing & Spoor, 1973).

While reports of such emissions had been associated with hearing disorders (see Dallos, 1981; Zurek, 1981), there has been some evidence that tonal generation occurs frequently in people with normal hearing. Zurek (1981) found that of 32 persons with normal hearing, 16 had acoustic emissions in one or both ears. In addition to these spontaneously generated sounds, stimulated acoustic emissions have been observed which consist of a delayed replica or acoustic echo generated by the ear following a brief stimulus. (See Dallos, 1981, for a review of this topic and its possible relation to other recent developments in cochlear physiology.)

Strong evidence for mechanical resonance of the stereocilia was reported for the alligator lizard by Peake and Ling (1980). Although the basilar papilla (the reptilian homologue of the basilar membrane) of the animal showed no traveling wave and no filtering characteristics when examined using the Mössbauer technique, there was a sharp frequency selectivity of hair cells and nerve fibers. Fettiplace and Crawford (1980) obtained intracellular recordings from single hair cells of another reptile (a turtle) and found sharp frequency selectivity. Cells were arranged tonotopically along the papilla, with sensitivity to the highest frequency found at the basal or stapedial end (as in mammals). However, as with the alligator lizard, there appeared to be no frequency selectivity of the structure supporting the hair cells, the hair cells appearing to behave in their temporal characteristics as would be expected for simple tuned resonators.

THE AUDITORY-ACOUSTIC PARADOX: EXCELLENT DISCRIMINATION FROM A POOR INSTRUMENT

Considered as an acoustical instrument, the construction and functioning of the ear is extremely poor. The ear is not unique in this respect; characteristics which could be considered as serious flaws in a physical instrument are found in other sensory systems as well. Thus, Helmholtz listed and described in some detail the optical defects of the normal eye which include severe spherical aberration, chromatic aberration, light scattering of colloidal particles, inhomogeneities suspended in the ocular fluids, and inside-out retinal design (the blood vessels and nerves are in front of the light-sensitive receptor cells and cast shadows, rather than being located behind the receptors as in the octopus eye). He then stated that, if an optician had tried to sell him an instrument with these defects, he would feel justified in blaming his carelessness in the strongest terms and returning the instrument (see Warren & Warren, 1968, pp. 73-80).

Comparable acoustical defects can be described for the performance of the ear. The pinna produces resonances and time delays which change the intensity and phase of spectral components in a manner which varies with azimuth and elevation of the source. The external ear canal operates as a resonant tube, selectively enhancing frequencies of about 3,000 or 4,000 Hz. The intra-aural muscles may have frequency selective effects when they contract. The acoustic system is known to introduce nonlinear distortions before neural transduction, so that sinusoidal stimuli at moderate intensity levels are associated with a variety of extraneous sinusoidal frequencies at the receptor level (see Dallos, 1981; Plomp, 1976).

Helmholtz pointed out that the optical imperfections of the eye were the consequence of a design no better than it absolutely had to be (or, as he put it, one doesn't use a razor to cut firewood). While optical defects may correspond to the limits of tolerable distortion in vision, it appears that some acoustical imperfections of the ear may serve actively to enhance auditory discrimination.

Although we can perceive relatively slight distortions and changes in spectral balance produced by loudspeakers and audio amplifiers, it is often impossible to detect the gross distortions and variations in spectral balance produced within our own ears. Acoustic distortions by the ear (which can be measured with appropriate techniques), if present consistently as part of the normal transduction process, are treated by the listener as nondistorted representations of the stimulus. Some acoustic transformations in spectral characteristics of a sound produced by pinna interaction, head shadows, etc. are associated with the spatial location of the source. (This will be discussed in some detail in chapter 2.) These position-dependent transformations do not interfere with identification of a sound, but do contribute to spatial localization. Thus, some spectral changes cannot be heard as such: they are transformed perceptually into differences in apparent location of a sound, with the sound itself seeming to remain unchanged.

ELECTROPHYSIOLOGICAL RESPONSE OF THE COCHLEA AND PERIPHERAL NEURAL APPARATUS

Most of our knowledge concerning the nature of neurophysiological processing of acoustic information deals with events occurring within cochlear structures and first order auditory neurons. We will deal first with the three types of electrical potentials generated by structures other than nerve fibers in the inner ear: the resting potential, the summating potential, and the cochlear microphonic.

The Resting Potential

In the absense of any stimulation by sound, DC (direct current) differences in resting potential are found between structures in the cochlea. Relative to the potential found for both perilymph and cortilymph, the endolymph of the scala media which bathes the stereocilia of the hair cells has a potential of +80 mV. Since the resting potential within the hair cells is about –70 mV, there is a very high potential difference (that is, for structures within the body) of 150 mV across the cell membrane at the stereocilia. Mechanical deformation of the stereocilia during stimulation by sound causes changes from the resting potential which eventuate in stimulation of neural fibers. The stria vascularis lining the scala media seems to be implicated in maintaining the high endo-lymph potential necessary for stimulation of the receptor cells.

The Summating Potential

When stimulation by sound occurs, there is a DC change from resting level, called the summating potential, which can be picked up by electrodes within and near the cochlea. The magnitude of the summating potential depends upon the location of the measuring electrode and the reference electrode, and it is generally greatest measured at the scala media. At any particular location, the summating potential appears to be a complex function of both sound frequency and sound intensity. Despite the fact that the summating potential was discovered some time ago (Davis, Fernandez, & McAuliffe, 1950), there is still considerable uncertainty concerning the details of its nature. But there is general agreement that there are a number of compo-nents and presumably different processes which summate to produce this potential.

The Cochlear Microphonic

The effect now called the cochlear microphonic was described by Wever and Bray in 1930. It was observed that if a sound was played in a cat's ear, an alternating current (AC) response could be picked up in the vicinity of the cochlea. When this AC response was amplified and played back through a loudspeaker, a fairly faithful copy of the stimulus was produced. Thus, when someone spoke into the cat's ear in one room, the amplified potential changes within the cat's cochlea could be played back by a loudspeaker in another room to produce a quite intelligible message. While Wever and Bray at first believed that they were measuring responses within the auditory nerve itself, Lord Adrian the following year (1931) reported some of his observations which indicated that a large part of the response measured by Wever and Bray was due to what he called the "cochlear microphonic," with only a small contribution attributable to potential changes within the auditory nerve. The cochlear microphonic can be picked up at positions some distance from the cochlea, although the position generally employed is near the round window. Figure 1.12 shows how closely the cochlear microphonic follows the acoustic stimulus. In making the trace of the cochlear microphonic shown in the figure, "difference" electrodes were used which were placed so as to make it possible to cancel out other types of potential changes. The cochlear microphonic appears without any latency (unlike neural responses), and the changes in the cochlear microphonic produced either by reduction of oxygen supply or introduction of anesthesia are different than the changes produced in neural activity. The frequency response limits of the cochlear microphonic to sinusoidal tones resemble the frequency limits of hearing of the animal under study, so that bats generate cochlear microphonics with frequencies well above the upper limits of response for man. Studies with animals have shown that, when hair cells with maximum sensitivity to particular frequencies are destroyed by prolonged exposure to intense tones of these frequencies,

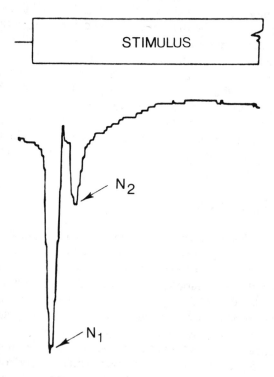

Fig. 1.13. Whole-nerve action potential response at the onset of a tone burst of 8,000 Hz. The tracing represents the average of the potentials within the scala vestibuli and the scala tympani. The time separating N_1 from N_2 depends upon the stimulus level, and is usually between 1 and 2 msec.
Source: From P. Dallos, *The Auditory Periphery: Biophysics and Physiology* (New York: Academic Press, 1973).

cochlear microphonic responses to these frequencies are abolished. Detailed investigations have shown that the integrity of the outer hair cells is required for normal cochlear microphonics, with inner hair cells playing a relatively minor role in the development of this response.

Whole Nerve Action Potential

When an electrode is placed near the cochlea and the indifferent or reference electrode at some remote site (such as the mouth or neck), the active electrode's response to sound reflects the effect of the whole nerve response as well as the summating potential and the cochlear microphonic. If the reference electrode is placed appropriately, various procedures are available which are capable of cancelling the potential changes attributable to summating potentials and cochlear microphonics (see Dallos, 1973). The isolated whole nerve action potential reflects the integrated activity of individual fibers. An example of this action potential is shown in figure 1.13. Usually, responses to clicks or to the onset of tone bursts are examined, since responses of individual nerve fibers consist of both negative and positive changes relative to their resting potential, and hence different nerve fibers can cancel each other when asynchronous responses are summed. Even with a click, the measured response is complicated by the fact that it may take some 3 msec for the traveling wave to move from base to apex of the cochlea, resulting in asynchronous responses, with some cancellation following the initial "pure" whole nerve response involving only fibers originating at the basal end. It is possible to obtain whole nerve action potentials in humans, and the information can be of diagnostic use in cases of hearing disorders.

Single Unit Receptor Potentials

The gross potential changes within the cochlea in response to sound which have been described above (summating potential, cochlear microphonic, whole nerve action potential) provide an environment in which further activity of single units in response to acoustic stimulation takes place. The first of these single unit responses to sound is the receptor potential. The auditory receptor cells terminate in stereocilia which, as we have seen, are bent by shearing forces when the traveling wave causes the basilar membrane to move relative to the tectorial membrane. This bending produces graded changes in receptor potential (that is, changes in magnitude which are monotonic functions of the angle of bending) which consist of both AC and DC components. The receptor potential acts upon the lower part of the receptor cell body containing presynaptic bars and possessing vesicles containing a chemical transmitter substance. Events associated with potential changes at the stereocilia cause release of this chemical transmitter which diffuses to the nearby endings of auditory nerve fibers, where changes induced in membrane permeability lead to a "generator potential" change in the fiber. (For further discussion of the distinction between receptor potential and generator potential, see Dallos, 1978; Davis, 1961, 1965.)

Single Unit Generator Potentials

The initial segment of the auditory nerve axon exhibits a graded potential change reflecting the receptor potential. The generator potential is conducted with a decrement (that is, the potential change from the resting or baseline level decreases with distance from the synaptic endings near the hair cells). After passing out through the habenula perforata, the unmyelinated axon gains a myelin sheath, and it appears to be at this region that the all-or-none action potential is generated. Neural events beyond this point are quantized (all-or-none) and conducted without decrement, as the result of metabolic processes within the nerve fiber, to the synaptic ending of this first order auditory neuron within the ipsilateral cochlear nucleus.

Action Potentials of Auditory Nerve Fibers

Using fine electrodes, it is possible to obtain responses from single fibers in the cochlear branch of the VIIIth nerve. Individual fibers have spontaneous discharge rates in the absence of sound varying from a few per second up to 100 per second or more. When the inner ear is stimulated by sound, the rate increases with intensity but cannot occur at rates greater than about 1,400 per second. The upper limit of response rate reflects the absolute refractory period (an interval during which the membrane potential increases in positive voltage while intracellular processes ready the neuron for further response). The neural discharge measured by an electrode appears as a voltage spike of fixed amplitude and corresponds to a potential change sweeping along the fiber from cochlea to cochlear nucleus.

Individual nerve fibers exhibit frequency selectivity reflecting their particular place of origin on the basilar membrane, and the sinusoidal frequency corresponding to their greatest sensitivity (lowest threshold) is called the best or characteristic frequency. Neurons with highest characteristic frequencies are found near the surface of the auditory nerve bundle, with characteristic frequency decreasing regularly toward the center.

The frequency selectivity of an auditory nerve fiber is often shown as a "tuning curve" in which the ordinate represents the threshold in dB and the abscissa the frequency of the stimulating tone. Figure 1.14 shows a number of tuning curves for individual auditory nerve fibers with different characteristic frequencies in a single cat. While the typical form of a tuning curve has a

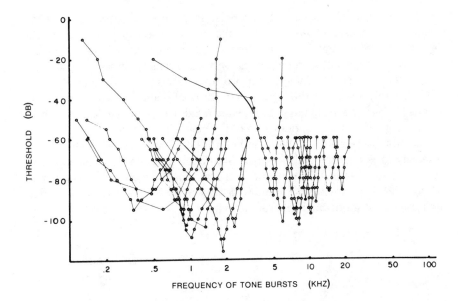

Fig. 1.14. Tuning curves of individual auditory nerve fibers with different characteristic frequencies in a single cat. Each curve represents the intensity in dB (relative to an arbitrary reference standard) needed to reach the response threshold of the fiber.
Source: From N.Y.-S. Kiang, *Discharge Patterns of Single Fibers in the Cat's Auditory Nerve*, Research Monograph No. 35 (Cambridge, Mass.: MIT Press, 1965). Reproduction by permission of the MIT Press.

gentle slope at the low frequency side of the characteristic frequency and a steep slope at the high frequency side, there are many other shapes. Some tuning curves are symmetrical, some have steeper slopes at the low frequency side, and a number of fibers show a break in the low frequency side of the tuning curve in which the slope becomes much less steep near the lower frequency limit of their response range. It seems that, while tuning curves reflect the general filter characteristics of the basilar membrane at the position of the receptor cells associated with nerve fibers, this correspondence between basilar membrane response and tuning curves is far from exact. One difference is that tuning curves are often sharper (have steeper slopes) than the filter characteristics of the basilar membrane. As discussed earlier, the shape of the tuning curve may reflect not only a frequency analysis corresponding to the basilar membrane displacements, but also the filter characteristics of stereocilia.

When the stimulus is raised to supraliminal levels, we can examine the "response area," or range of frequencies and amplitudes to which a fiber responds. One useful measure within the response area is the response rate (spikes/sec) of a single fiber measured for different frequencies at a fixed dB level, with the process repeated at various intensity levels. These "iso-intensity contours" for a single fiber of a squirrel monkey are shown in figure 1.15. It can be seen in this figure that not only does contour change with intensity, but the frequency producing maximal response also changes. Considering only the response rate of the single fiber shown in this figure, it would not be possible to tell whether the stimulus were a relatively low intensity tone near the characteristic frequency or a relatively high intensity tone at a greater distance from the characteristic frequency. However, a single fiber may provide information identifying particular frequencies within its response area through phase-locking.

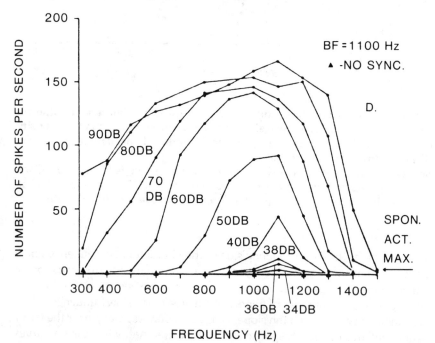

Fig. 1.15. Iso-intensity contours for a single fiber of a squirrel monkey. The characteristic frequency or best frequency (BF) of this fiber is 1,100 Hz. The arrow to the right of the figure indicates the level of spontaneous activity, and the triangular data points indicate the low level of activity at which there is no phase-locking of spikes to the stimulus waveform.

Source: From J.E. Rose, J.E. Hind, D.J. Anderson, and J.F. Brugge, "Some Effects of Stimulus Intensity on Response of Auditory Nerve Fibers in the Squirrel Monkey," *Journal of Neurophysiology* 34 (1971): 685-99.

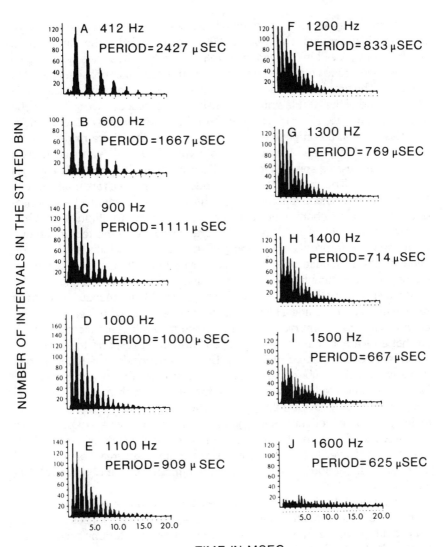

TIME IN MSEC.

Fig. 1.16. Interval histograms from a single nerve fiber in a squirrel monkey. The abscissa gives the interval between successive spikes, with resolution into bins of 100 μsec duration. Dots below the abscissa indicate integral multiples of the period for each frequency. For further details, see text.

Source: From J.E. Rose, J.F. Brugge, D.J. Anderson, and J.E. Hind, "Phase-locked Response to Low-Frequency Tones in Single Auditory Nerve Fibers of the Squirrel Monkey," *Journal of Neurophysiology* 30 (1967): 769-73.

Response spikes of the fiber tend to be locked to a particular phase angle of a sinusoidal stimulus. Thus, when a 200 Hz tone is used as the stimulus, and this frequency is within the response area of a single fiber, spikes picked up by the microelectrodes may be synchronous with a particular phase-angle of the stimulus. The time between successive neural spikes is some integral multiple of the period of the 200 Hz sinusoid (5 msec), so that successive spikes can be separated by 5, 10, 15, or more msec. An individual nerve fiber generally does not discharge in a completely regular manner, so that there might be a 10 msec interval followed by a 20 msec interval followed by a 5 msec interval between successive spikes. However, if a recording of the pattern of firing is examined, it will be apparent that all periods between spikes are multiples of a 5 msec period. The phenomenon of phase-locking seems to be a consequence of the mechanics of cochlear events leading to stimulation. Only upward movement of the basilar membrane relative to the tectorial membrane appears to produce a bending of the stereocilia which is effective in initiating the sequence of events leading to neural stimulation. As the frequency of the stimulating sinusoid is increased, phase-locking can be observed up to about 4,000 or 5,000 Hz as long as the frequency is within the response area of the fiber. However, as has been pointed out earlier, fibers cannot discharge at intervals shorter than roughly 700 μsec (microseconds), so that above about 1,400 Hz, a single fiber cannot respond to successive statements of a repeated waveform. But, if we consider the whole nerve, there will be some fibers responding to each repetition of the waveform. Hence, as suggested by Wever (1949), the rate at which "volleys" of neural firing occur can provide information concerning tonal frequency. Phase-locking is not exact, and some jitter occurs which, when expressed as microsecond deviations from exact phase-locking, becomes less at high frequencies. Nevertheless, the variability becomes so great for a sinusoid near 4,000 Hz (period of 250 μsec) that the temporal smear obscures phase-locking.

The extent of phase-locking can be shown by interspike interval histograms. The histogram shown in figure 1.16 is based on responses of a single fiber to a tone of the frequency shown when presented for one second for a total of 10 times. The abscissa shows the time between successive spikes (discharges) of a single auditory fiber, and the ordinate the total number of occurrences of interspike intervals with this value. The same phase angle of the sinusoid occurs at integral multiples of the sinusoid's period, and it can be seen that responses tended to occur at integral multiples of the particular period of the stimulus tone. For example, at 412 Hz, the periods between successive spikes generally were integral multiples of the tonal period of 2,427 μsec (the time required for a single cycle of the 412 Hz tone), with more responses occurring at a value equal to the tonal period than for any multiple of this value.

2

Spatial Localization and Binaural Hearing

In the previous chapter it was noted that the ear modifies and distorts the acoustic signal before it reaches the receptor cells, and that changes which would be considered defects if produced by microphones or other physical instruments can furnish valuable perceptual information. Thus, the complex acoustic changes produced by the pinnae when a source moves, provide information concerning position, and result in perception of an unchanging sound at a changing location. In this chapter, we will discuss the effects produced by the pinnae, as well as other examples of how changes in acoustic input are not perceived as differences in the nature of the sound, but rather as differences in position.

Obviously, it often is important for us to know the position of a sound source, but there is another advantage associated with the ability to localize sound. As we shall see, mechanisms employed for localization allow us to hear signals which would otherwise be inaudible.

Any position in space can be specified relative to an observer by its azimuth (angle from straight ahead measured in the horizontal plane), elevation (angle from the horizontal measured in a vertical plane), and distance. Unfortunately, it is difficult to study localization of sound sources in space using headphones because the sounds generated by them usually have apparent sources within the listener's head (for reasons which will be discussed subsequently). These intracranial images can be made to move to the right or left by appropriate differences in the stimuli delivered to each ear, but such lateral images do not have a specific azimuth as do externalized sound images. It is conventional to use the term "lateralization" to describe intracranial sidedness of sound images produced through headphones, and "localization" to describe positioning of externalized images. The localization of a source in space involves both binaural (dichotic) cues based upon differences in the input to each ear, and monaural cues for which the stimulus to one ear alone can provide information concerning location of the source.

BINAURAL PERCEPTION OF AZIMUTH

In 1876 and 1877, Lord Rayleigh demonstrated that lateral positions of complex sounds such as voices could be identified accurately, as could high frequency sinusoidal tones. He attributed this localization ability to interaural intensity differences caused by the head's sound shadow. It was not until some 30 years later that Rayleigh (1907) appreciated that interaural phase differences also could be used for determining the lateral position of low frequency pure tones. He proposed at that time his influential "duplex" theory which considered that high frequencies are located laterally by inter-aural intensity differences while low frequencies are located laterally by interaural phase (or time) differences.

Figure 2.1 shows the analysis of Woodworth (1938) of how interaural path-length differences (leading to interaural time and phase differences) arise when a source is to the right or left of the medial plane. This figure shows the additional path length as due to two segments: a straight line portion, d_1, and the curved portion following the contour of the skull, d_2. The total increase in path distance, ΔD to the further ear is described by the expression:

$$\Delta D = d_1 + d_2 = r(\theta + \sin\theta) \qquad \text{(Eq. 1)}$$

where r is the radius of the head considered as a circle, and θ is the azimuth of a distant source measured in radians. This formula can be converted to give values for time delay, ΔT. If we consider that the radius of the head is 8.5 cm, and the speed of sound is 34,000 cm/sec, then the difference in time of arrival of sound at the two ears is given by the expression:

$$\Delta T = 250(\theta + \sin\theta) \text{ msec.} \qquad \text{(Eq. 2)}$$

Interaural phase differences are unambiguous cues to azimuth only at low frequencies. When a sinusoidal tone is about 650 Hz, its wavelength (about 50 cm) corresponds to about twice the path-length increment to the further ear with sources at azimuths of 90° or 270° from the medial plane. Hence, there will be a 180° interaural phase difference (that is, a pressure peak in one ear will occur at the same time as a pressure trough in the other) whether the source is at 90° or 270°. When the sinusoidal frequencies are higher than about 1,300 Hz, multiple ambiguities occur with several azimuth angles corresponding to the same interaural phase difference, and phase no longer is a useful indicator of azimuth for sinusoidal tones.

Woodworth's model has been tested directly by measuring time differen-ces for the arrival of clicks at the two ears (Feddersen, Sandel, Teas, & Jeffress, 1957), as shown in figure 2.2. It can be seen that the values obtained agree very well with Woodworth's model. However, measurements using sinusoidal tones (see Abbagnaro, Bauer, & Torick, 1975; Kuhn, 1977) have indicated that Woodworth's assumption that interaural time delays (ITDs) are independent of frequency of tones is incorrect, especially for low frequencies, apparently due to interactions with sound diffracted by the head. Roth, Kochhar, and Hind (1980) have suggested that there might be two kinds of ITDs, one which they called "steady state" ITD and another which they called "group" ITD. They hypothesized that each of these time delays might be encoded by separate groups of neurons.

There have been direct measures of detection thresholds for interaural

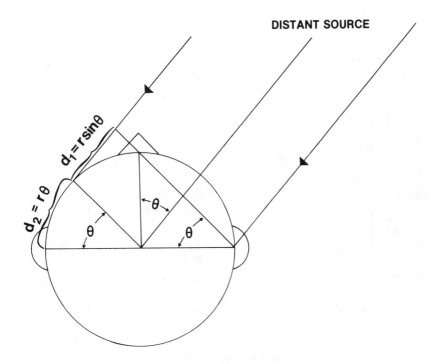

Fig. 2.1. Path-length difference between the two ears corresponding to the azimuth of the source, θ. The additional distance to the further ear is shown as the sum of a straight line segment, d_1, and a curved segment following the contour of the head, d_2. The path-length difference can be used to calculate the difference in time of arrival of sound at the two ears, as described in the text. The effects of the pinnae are not considered in this model.

Source: Adapted from R.S. Woodworth, *Experimental Psychology* (New York: Holt, 1938).

time differences using sinusoidal tones of different frequencies delivered through headphones. Klumpp and Eady (1956) determined the minimal time delay permitting listeners to lateralize a sound correctly to the side of the leading ear 75 percent of the time. A minimum of about 10 μsec was found for a 1,000 Hz tone (this time difference corresponds to an azimuth of about 2° for an external source). The threshold rose to 24 μsec at 1,300 Hz, and was not measurable (i.e., phase differences could not be detected at all) at 1,500 Hz and above. When frequencies were decreased from 1,000 Hz, there was a regular increase in interaural delay thresholds, reaching 75 μsec at 90 Hz (the lowest frequency used).

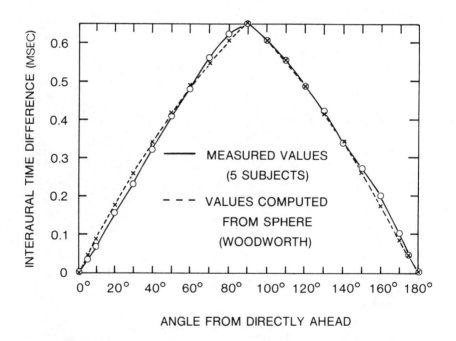

ANGLE FROM DIRECTLY AHEAD

Fig. 2.2. Interaural time differences for clicks as a function of azimuth. The solid line connects values as measured at the ears of actual heads, and the dashed line connects values calculated by Woodworth's procedure for a spherical head.

Source: Adapted from W.E. Feddersen, T.T. Sandel, D.C. Teas, and L.A. Jeffress, "Localization of High-Frequency Tones," *Journal of the Acoustical Society of America* 29 (1957): 988-91.

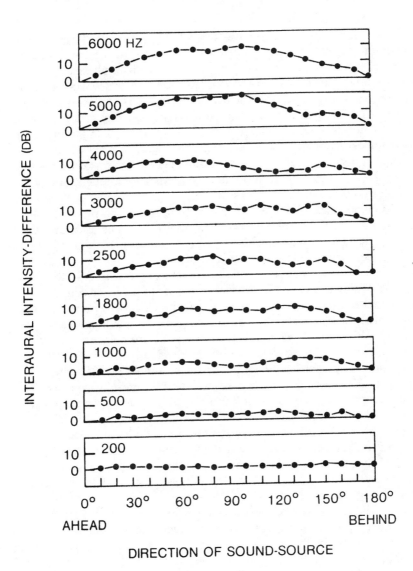

Fig. 2.3. Interaural intensity differences measured as a function of azimuth for sinusoidal tones of different frequencies. It can be seen that there is no appreciable sound shadow cast by the head at 200 Hz, and a considerable shadow cast by the head at 6,000 Hz. The lack of symmetry in the front quadrant (0° to 90°) relative to the rear quadrant (90° to 180°) is attributable to the pinna.

Source: Adapted from W.E. Feddersen, T.T. Sandel, D.C. Teas, and L.A. Jeffress, "Localization of High-Frequency Tones," *Journal of the Acoustical Society of America* 29 (1957): 988-91.

As mentioned earlier, Rayleigh's duplex theory considered that sources of high frequency sounds can be located laterally through interaural intensity differences, so that when frequency becomes too high for phase to operate, intensity comes into play. When a sphere has a diameter which is greater than roughly half the wavelength of a sinusoidal tone, it will cast an appreciable sound shadow. The head casts such a shadow, resulting in a detectable interaural intensity difference starting at about 1,000 Hz, with the interaural intensity difference increasing with frequency. Figure 2.3 shows measurements by Feddersen, Sandel, Teas, and Jeffress (1957) of interaural intensity differences as a function of the azimuth of the source for frequencies ranging from 200 to 6,000 Hz. Were the head a sphere without pinnae, the curves would be symmetrical about 90°. However, the pinnae do produce sound shadows and resonances for high frequency tones (as will be discussed later) which enter into the asymmetries seen in this figure.

The accuracy of listeners' estimates of the azimuth of a loudspeaker producing pure tones was measured by Stevens and Newman (1936). Subjects were seated in a chair elevated above a roof to minimize sound reflections and approximate an anechoic (echo-free) environment, and measurements were made early in the morning to reduce extraneous sounds. When tone bursts (as well as noise and clicks) were delivered at various azimuths, a sizable number of front-back reversals were noted (that is, sources on the same side differing by the same number of degrees from 90° were confused), but confusions of right and left were almost never made. The greatest errors occurred at about 3,000 Hz, with error scores dropping at higher and lower frequencies. In a more recent experiment, Sandel, Teas, Feddersen, and Jeffress (1955) used listeners seated in an anechoic room with head movements restricted by use of a clamp. Broad-band noise and sinusoidal tones were heard alternately, each fading in and out gradually to minimize transient clicks. The broad-band noise was used as an acoustic pointer, being adjusted to correspond to the apparent azimuth of the tone. Sandel and his colleagues (1955) reported a lower value (about 1,500 Hz) for the frequency producing poorest accuracy in localization than did Stevens and Newman. As in the earlier study, front-back confusions were quite common. This is not surprising if we consider that the interaural time delays are equivalent for such positions. The question that needs answering seems to be how discrimination between positions in the front quadrant and the back quadrant can be made at all.

There appear to be two main ways in which front-back errors can be minimized when dealing with real sources in everyday life: one involves asymmetrical effects of the pinna which will be discussed subsequently, and the other involves head movements. Changes in time of arrival correlated with lateral head-turning can disambiguate the direction of continuing sounds. For example, if the sound is on the right side, rotation of the head to the right will decrease the interaural time difference for sources in the front quadrant and will increase the interaural time difference for sources in the back quadrant.

Minimal Audible Angle

Mills (1958, 1972) measured the minimum angle permitting lateral resolution of tones, calling it the minimal audible angle by analogy to the well-known minimum visual angle. Listeners sat in an anechoic chamber with the position of their head fixed by a restraining clamp. Pairs of sinusoidal tone pulses were presented, and listeners were requested to tell whether the second pulse

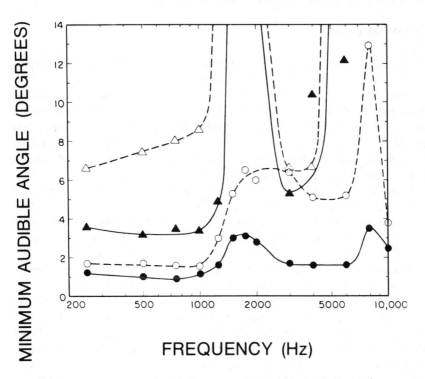

Fig. 2.4. The minimum audible angle between successive pulses of a tone as a function of the frequency of the tone and the azimuth of the source (● = 0°; ○= 30°; ▲ = 60°; △ = 75°).

Source: From A.W. Mills, "Auditory Localization," in J.V. Tobias (Ed.), *Foundations of Modern Auditory Theory.* Vol. 2 (New York: Academic Press, 1972), pp. 303-48.

came from the right or left of the first (the source was moved in the short interval separating the pulses). Figure 2.4 shows the results obtained. The minimal audible angle is the least when measured as variation from 0 degrees (straight ahead). Since listeners tend to orient toward the source of a sound of interest, the source is usually brought into the region of most accurate localization. Also, it often is possible to visually fixate a sound source near the medial plane, so that interaural cues to localization can be calibrated against the more accurate visual localization. In the medial plane, the minimum auditory angle is about one degree for high and low frequencies, being greater for frequencies from 1,500 to 2,000 Hz. (The minimum discriminable visual angle is about one minute.) The high minimum auditory angle at midrange frequencies is in keeping with the duplex theory considering that judgments of azimuth are based on interaural phase differences at low frequencies and interaural intensity differences at high frequencies.

Binaural Beats

When tones are mistuned slightly from unison and introduced separately into the two ears, binaural beats may be observed which are characterized by changing localization or fluctuation in intensity. For example, if a tone of 500 Hz is presented to one ear and 500.5 Hz to the other, a listener may hear a phantom source which moves from side to side, with lateralization associated with leading phase. Intensity maxima may also occur with beats slower than one per second, but they are not very noticeable and show no consistent relation to phase angle. For fast beat rates (a few per second), lateralization shifts become difficult to hear, and listeners generally report an intensity fluctuation having a diffuse intracranial location (Lane, 1925). The upper frequency limit for the production of binaural beats by sinusoidal tones is uncertain. These beats are generally considered to be strongest for frequencies from about 300 to 600 Hz, becoming difficult to hear at 1,000 Hz. However, Wever (1949) claimed that by using "very slight frequency differences" he was able to obtain binaural beats (or lateralization shifts) up to 3,000 Hz. Wever also referred to an unpublished study by Loesch and Kapell indicating that subjects could hear binaural beats up to 2,500 Hz after about 10 hours of practice. Since there was evidence of increasing frequency limits with increasing practice time at the end of the experiment, Wever stated that "it seems certain" that further improvement would have occurred with further practice. It appears that the extent of practice and frequency separation (or beat rate) employed could be responsible for much of the variability in reports from different laboratories concerning the upper frequency limit for binaural beats.

Binaural beats were of importance in the development of the duplex theory of sound localization, since they helped convince Lord Rayleigh (1907) that interaural phase differences could indeed be detected. Rayleigh's earlier doubts appear to have been based upon the observation of Helmholtz and others that changing the phase relations between harmonic components of complex tones delivered to the same ear generally could *not* be detected.

Thus far, we have been considering the effect of time-of-arrival delays upon perception of laterality for sinusoidal tones. Rather different results are obtained when either clicks or continuing complex sounds are used.

Detection of Interaural Delays for Clicks and for Complex Sounds

Klumpp and Eady (1956) obtained thresholds for detection of interaural time differences using a delay line to deliver a variety of different sounds through headphones. We have already discussed their report that the lowest threshold value of 10 μsec was obtained with a 1,000 Hz tone, with the detection of time delay becoming impossible at frequencies of 1,500 Hz and above. When they presented a single 1 μsec click, a delay threshold of 28 μsec was found, but a 2 sec burst consisting of 30 such clicks had a delay threshold of only 11 μsec, indicating that integration of information from the individual clicks of a burst took place. When broad-band noise was used, a threshold value of 10 μsec was found, with approximately the same threshold observed for a 150-1,700 Hz noise band. Other noise bands with different bandwidths and frequency ranges had somewhat higher thresholds.

It might be thought that spectral frequency components of noise lying below 1,500 Hz were required for detection of time differences, since Klumpp and Eady had found that phase differences for sinusoidal tones of 1,500 Hz and above were ineffective in producing any lateralization. As discussed in chapter 1, low frequency tones produce a phase-locking of neural response, so that an interaural temporal comparison of fibers with the same low characteristic frequencies locked to the same phase angle could provide the temporal information for lateralization of broad-band noise. However, Klumpp and Eady found that a narrow-band noise containing frequencies from about 3,000 to 3,300 Hz could be lateralized (although the threshold was at the fairly high value of 60 μsec). It would appear that temporal information carried by the high frequency noise could be used for lateralization, despite the widely held duplex theory considering that temporal information is restricted to low frequency spectral components. Henning (1974) provided an interesting demonstration of the nature of this temporal information. He introduced interaural time delays using a 3,900 Hz tone amplitude-modulated at 300 Hz (that is, the intensity of a 3,900 Hz tone was varied in a sinusoidal fashion 300 times a second). Henning found that interaural time delays in the amplitude modulation pattern could be detected with this stimulus at approximately the same threshold delay as found for a 300 Hz sinusoidal tone, despite the absence of any low frequency spectral components (spectrally, this amplitude modulated stimulus can be considered as consisting of three sinusoidal frequencies of 3,600, 3,900, and 4,200 Hz). It appears to be the time pattern of intensity changes in the high frequency carrier tone (or its "envelope") which is compared interaurally. McFadden and Pasanen (1975) used binaural beats to provide another demonstration that complex waveforms consisting of tones well above the classical limit of 1,000 Hz could give rise to dichotic temporal interactions. When a 3,000 Hz tone was presented to both ears and mixed with a 3,100 Hz tone at the left ear and a 3,101 Hz tone at the right ear, the difference in the interaural envelope frequencies (100 vs. 101 Hz) produced binaural beating at a rate of one per second. Binaural beats were noted even when the spectral components in the two ears were rather different as long as the envelopes were close in frequency: thus 2,000 and 2,050 Hz in one ear would cause binaural beats of 1/sec when heard with 3,000 and 3,051 Hz in the other ear.

DETECTION OF LONG INTERAURAL DELAYS

Most experiments dealing with the limits for detection of interaural temporal delay have studied the lower limit (the shortest detectable delay). But where does the upper limit lie? As we shall see, this limit is surprisingly high—at least one-half second for broad-band noise delivered first to one ear and then to the other. At these long interaural delays, the sound is no longer lateralized to the leading ear.

As we increase the interaural delay for broad-band noise from the threshold of about 10 μsec reported by Klumpp and Eady, we perceive an increase in the extent of lateralization of the fused single image up to delays of several hundred microseconds. The greatest possible delay attributable to interaural path-length differences is roughly 650 μsec, and as would be expected, listeners hear a single lateral source at this delay. However, if the delay is increased to about 2,000 μsec (2 msec), this sharp single lateral image starts to become diffuse (Bilsen & Goldstein, 1974). Blodgett, Wilbanks, and Jeffress (1956) reported that sidedness is lost for broad-band noise with interaural delays of about 9.5 msec. The delay range producing diffuse lateralization is of interest because it appears possible to hear either lateralization to the leading ear or a pitch equivalent to that of a sinusoidal tone of $1/\tau$ Hz (where τ is the time delay in sec), but not both. Fourcin (1965, 1970) used a variety of stimuli which permitted his listeners to hear this interaural delay pitch. The simplest condition involved broad-band noise from two generators delivered to each ear: the noise from one generator was presented diotically (identical presentation in each ear), while the noise from the second generator had an interaural delay of a few milliseconds. Fourcin found that an interaural delay of τ sec produced a pitch matching that of a sinusoidal tone of $1/\tau$ Hz. Later, Bilsen and Goldstein (1974) reported that it was possible to hear a faint pitch of $1/\tau$ Hz with noise from only a single source delivered to one ear several msec after delivery to the other. (Pitches were produced for delays ranging from about 3×10^{-3} through 1.2×10^{-2} sec, corresponding to 333 and 85 Hz respectively.) Warren, Bashford, and Wrightson (1981) confirmed Bilsen and Goldstein's findings, but found that their subjects had a somewhat greater delay limit for the production of pitch (5×10^{-2} sec delay corresponding to a pitch of 20 Hz). But, in addition, Warren and his colleagues (1981) reported that an infrapitch periodicity could be detected at considerably longer interaural delays, down to a lower limit of 0.5 sec (corresponding to a repetition time of about 2 Hz). These long delay periods could be matched in repetition time with periodic pulses delivered simultaneously to both ears (as could pitch-range interaural delays). In addition, for delays greater than 200 msec (corresponding to 5 Hz) the repetition period could be matched by finger tapping without the need for matching to a second auditory stimulus. As we shall see in chapter 3, repetition of diotically delivered noise also can be perceived at 2 Hz, and the ability to detect long period repetition has implications for theories concerning neural periodicity analysis.

Interestingly, although listeners could detect long interaural delays, they could not tell which ear received the noise first. After perception of laterality was lost for delays greater than roughly 10 msec, the noise was heard as a spatial blur positioned symmetrically about the medial plane, and repetition was perceived as occurring within this space regardless of which ear received the noise first. A similar indefinite location has been reported for uncorrelated noises with equivalent long-term spectral characteristics delivered to each ear (David, Guttman, & van Bergeijk, 1958; Kock, 1950; Warren & Bashford, 1976). Thus, while fusion into a single image does not take place either with long interaural delays of noise or with uncorrelated noises presented to each ear, neither is there an ability to hear two lateral inputs.

The following section deals with other examples of the loss of lateralization of monaural signals induced by contralateral sounds, and discusses evidence indicating that processing leading to delateralization corresponds to an early stage in auditory localization.

CONTRALATERAL INDUCTION

There have been several reports that monaural sounds seem to shift away from the stimulated side in the presence of qualitatively different sounds delivered to the other ear. Using headphones, Egan (1948) found monaural speech to be displaced toward the side of a contralateral noise, and Thurlow and Elfner (1959) found that a monaural tone would be "pulled in" toward the contralateral ear when it received a monaural tone of different frequency. Related pulling effects were found by Butler and Naunton (1962, 1964) when they stimulated listeners simultaneously with a monaural headphone and a moveable loudspeaker. Warren and Bashford (1976) considered that the shift in localization of a monaural sound induced by a qualitatively different contralateral sound provided a method for investigating the limiting conditions for binaural interactions. They developed a procedure for delateralizing a monaural signal completely using a contralateral noise of appropriate spectral composition and intensity, and found that this delateralization (which they called "contralateral induction") required that the noise have a spectrum and intensity such that the signal could be present as a masked component within the noise. Thus, operating in everyday life, contralateral induction can prevent mislocalization of a source heard in one ear, but masked by an extraneous sound in the other. In addition, it appears that contralateral induction represents a general early stage in binaural processing.

The monaural signals used in the contralateral induction experiments were presented to one ear and a noise to the other, with the sides receiving signal and noise reversing each 500 msec, as shown in figure 2.5. The noise was always at 80 dB SPL, and the listener could adjust the level of the signal.

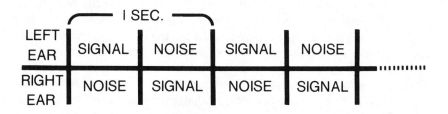

Fig. 2.5. Alternating pattern of dichotic stimulation used to produce delateralization of the signal through contralateral induction.
Source: From R.M. Warren and J.A. Bashford, "Auditory Contralateral Induction: An Early Stage in Binaural Processing," *Perception & Psychophysics* 20 (1976): 380-86.

For levels below the upper limit for contralateral induction, the monaural signal appeared to be stationary at a diffusely defined position symmetrical about the medial plane, while the noise was heard to switch from side to side each 500 msec. If the signal intensity was raised above the limit of contralateral induction, an abrupt change took place and the signal (as well as the noise) was heard to switch from side to side. Figure 2.6 shows the upper limit of contralateral induction for tones from 200 through 8,000 Hz when alternated with: (1) broad-band white noise; (2) one-third octave narrow-band noise centered at 1,000 Hz (slopes of 32 dB/octave); (3) band-reject white noise with a one-octave wide rejected band centered at 1,000 Hz (slopes of 80 dB/octave). It can be seen that curves for contralateral induction of the tones follow the spectral content of the contralateral noise, being relatively flat for the broad-band noise, rising to a maximum at 1,000 Hz for the narrow-band noise, and showing a minimum at the frequencies of the missing band for the band-reject noise. Figure 2.7, from the same study, shows contralateral induction limits for narrow-band filtered speech with center frequencies of 1,000 Hz and 3,000 Hz (bandwidth one-third octave, slopes 48 dB/octave) when presented with a contralateral one-third octave band noise at the center frequencies shown (slopes 32 dB/octave). It can be seen that, as with tonal signals, contralateral induction for narrow-band speech was maximum when the noise contained the same frequencies as the signals. As a consequence of this study, Warren and Bashford suggested the following rule: "If the peri-

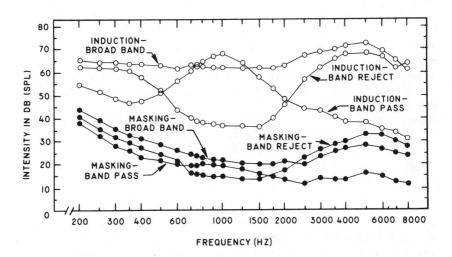

Fig. 2.6. Upper intensity limit for delateralization (contralateral induction) of monaural tones presented with one of three contralateral 80 dB SPL noises: broad-band noise; narrow-band (band-pass) noise centered at 1,000 Hz; and band-reject noise (rejected frequency band centered at 1,000 Hz). The detection thresholds in the presence of each type of noise are shown as well, and the differences betweeen these masked detection thresholds and the upper limit of induction represent the range of intensities over which delateralization of the tones occurred.

Source: From R.M. Warren and J.A. Bashford, "Auditory Contralateral Induction: An Early Stage in Binaural Processing," *Perception & Psychophysics* 20 (1976): 380-86.

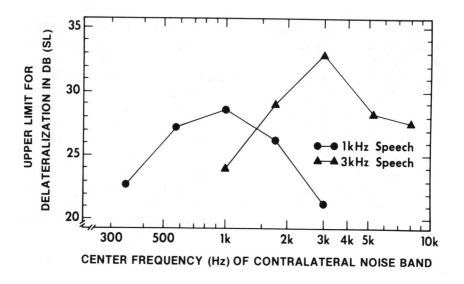

Fig. 2.7. Upper intensity limit for delateralization (contralateral induction) of monaural filtered speech bands centered at 1,000 Hz and 3,000 Hz when presented with contralateral 80 dB SPL narrow-band noises of various center frequencies. Intensity of speech is given as sensation level (dB above threshold).

Source: From R.M. Warren and J.A. Bashford, "Auditory Contralateral Induction: An Early Stage in Binaural Processing," *Perception & Psychophysics* 20 (1976): 380-86.

pheral neural units stimulated on the side receiving the louder noise include those corresponding to an ongoing contralateral signal, the fainter signal is released from lateralization and moves to a diffuse position located symmetrically about the medial plane." When they used the same procedure for alternating the sides receiving signal and noise (see Fig. 2.5) but employed as the "signal" noise of the same spectral characteristics at a level 1 dB below that of the uncorrelated contralateral "noise," an interesting effect was observed. There was a continuous diffusely localized noise centered on the medial plane (as described earlier for uncorrelated noises presented to each ear); but, in addition, a faint second noise was perceived off to the side which was receiving the stronger signal. The apparent intensity of this second sound was determined by the difference in sound pressure level of the noise presented to each ear, and appeared to be the consequence of the subtractive nature of contralateral induction; that is, in achieving delateralization of a monaural signal, corresponding components are subtracted from the input to the other ear.

It was suggested that contralateral induction might correspond to an early stage common to all types of binaural interaction associated with sound localization. This stage involves a cross-ear comparison of power spectra which determines whether a sound present at one ear could be present at the other ear as well; if so, the sound is released from lateralization. The further processing of binaural input required to produce sharply localized images of external sources involves such factors as: (1) appropriate relative intensities at the two ears for each of the spectral components corresponding to a single source at a particular location; (2) appropriate phase or time-of-arrival relations at the two ears corresponding to the analysis described under (1); and (3) changes in (1) and (2) correlated with head movements.

It should be noted that these experiments dealing with contralateral induction have employed the simplest possible arrangement for dichotic interaction: only one sound at each ear. A number of other studies have employed more complex stimulus arrangements.

If separate sounds are introduced to each ear (as in contralateral induction experiments), but in addition one of these sounds is introduced to the other ear as well (i.e., one sound is monaural and the other diotic), or if each of the two sounds is delivered to both ears with interaural phase or time-of-arrival differences for at least one of these sounds, then processing beyond the stage of contralateral induction becomes possible leading to "masking level differences." This topic has been the subject of much investigation.

MASKING LEVEL DIFFERENCES

Irving Langmuir, a Nobel laureate in chemistry, was the leader of a wartime project on the detection of sonar signals in noise. He and his associates noted that, when a tone and a masking noise appeared to be located at different azimuths because of binaural phase (or time-of-arrival) differences, the tone could be heard at levels as much as 15 dB below the limit of detectability found in the absence of directional differences between signal and noise (Langmuir, Schaefer, Ferguson, & Hennelly, 1944). Hirsh (1948a, 1948b) independently made a similar discovery, and undertook the first systematic study of this effect which came to be known as "masking level differences" (MLDs). In order to deal with Hirsh's studies and the many subsequent studies using a great variety of conditions, it is convenient to use a conventional system of notation: "S" denotes the signal, "M" is used for the masker, and subscripts are employed to indicate the relative interaural phase of S and M, with the subscript "o" used for no phase difference, and the subscript "π" for "antiphasic" or 180° phase difference. The subscript "u" is used with M to designate uncorrelated noise in each ear (that is, noise matched in long-term spectrum, but from independent sources). Some conditions used for S and M are summarized below:

S_o : Signal presented binaurally with no interaural differences.

M_o : Masker presented binaurally with no interaural differences.

S_m : Signal presented to only one ear.

M_m : Masker presented to only one ear.

S_π : Signal presented to one ear 180° out-of-phase relative to the signal presented to the other ear.

M_π : Masker presented to one ear 180° out-of-phase relative to the masker presented to the other ear.

M_u : Maskers presented to the two ears consisting of uncorrelated noise having the same long-term spectrum.

Green and Yost (1975) summarized the typical experimental findings obtained over the years in table 2.1, which is based on the use of a loud continuous broad-band noise as M, and a 500 Hz sinusoid for brief durations (10-100 msec) as S. The values listed for MLDs represent the differences in masked thresholds for the tone under the reference condition $S_m M_m$ (signal and masker mixed and heard monaurally in the same ear) and the conditions specified in the table.

Table 2.1. Masking level differences (MLDs) for various interaural differences

Interaural Condition	MLD (Compared to $M_m S_m$)
$M_\pi S_\pi$, $M_o S_o$, $M_u S_m$	0 dB
$M_u S_\pi$	3 dB
$M_u S_o$	4 dB
$M_\pi S_m$	6 dB
$M_o S_m$	9 dB
$M_\pi S_o$	13 dB
$M_o S_\pi$	15 dB

Source: From D. M. Green and W. A. Yost, "Binaural Analysis," in W.D. Keidel and W.D. Neff (Eds.), *Handbook of Sensory Physiology*. Vol. 2 (Berlin: Springer-Verlag, 1975), pp. 461-80.

MLD studies generally use noise as M and sinusoidal tones, speech, or pulse trains as S. Most studies have dealt with tonal signals, and it has been found that MLDs for tones decrease above 500 or 1,000 Hz, and for $M_\pi S_o$ and $M_o S_\pi$ reach asymptotic values of about 3 dB above 1,500 Hz. Over the years, a considerable number of theories have been proposed for MLDs (for review, see Green, 1976), some of which involve mechanisms employed for lateralization. There is good reason to believe that lateralization and MLDs are closely related, since differences in apparent position of S and M are necessary for generation of MLDs.

While MLDs involve the use of headphones, a similar very sizable reduction in the masked threshold occurs under normal listening conditions involving sources positioned in space when a signal originating at one location is subject to interference from other sounds at other locations. The spatial separation of sound images resulting from binaural differences in acoustic input can allow us to hear signals which would otherwise be masked, as demonstrated by the increased intelligibility observed for stereo relative to one-channel recordings of speech under noisy conditions. The so-called "cocktail party effect," which permits us to attend to one of several competing conversations, depends in part on the ability to concentrate on voices originating at one particular location.

TWO TYPES OF TEMPORAL DISPARITY

Tobias and Schubert (1959) compared the effects of different types of temporal disparity on lateralization. Short bursts of noise from 10 to 1,000 msec were used which could be gated to produce interaural onset disparities of 0 to 400 msec. The noise was passed through a delay line to produce a temporal disparity in fine structure which could be placed in opposition to the onset disparity (i.e., the ear hearing the noise first would have fine structure correspondence occurring later). Each cue operating alone (either onset disparity or fine structure disparity) could produce lateralization of short noise bursts to whichever side led in time. Subjects were required to adjust the fine structure disparity to cancel onset disparity so that the image was brought to the center of the head. As the noise burst durations were increased from 10 msec, briefer fine structure disparity was needed to offset the onset disparity. At the longer burst durations (300 msec or more), the onset disparity was of little importance for centering judgments, which were based essentially on fine structure.

Hafter, Dye, and Gilkey (1979) studied the ability of listeners to lateralize a tone on the basis of phase differences in the absence of onset and offset disparities. The transients corresponding to the beginning and end of the tonal signals were masked by noise, so that only the interaural phase differen-ces of the tones could be used for lateralization. It was found that when duration of the tone was sufficient for it to escape being masked by the preceding and following noise, excellent lateralization performance was observed on the basis of phase or fine structure alone. Kunov and Abel (1981) eliminated transient cues in a different manner by using slow rise/decay times of their tonal signals. They found that rise/decay times of at least 200 msec were necessary to obtain lateralization judgments based solely upon phase.

While these studies have dealt with different types of temporal cues to lateralization, another class of experiments has dealt with "time-intensity trading" in which time and intensity cues to sidedness were put in opposition.

TIME-INTENSITY TRADING

It is possible to have interaural time differences indicate that a sound is on one side while interaural intensity differences indicate the sound is on the other side. (This occurs when the side leading in time receives the fainter sound.) Among the early workers measuring the msec per dB required to produce a centered image with conflicting cues were Shaxby and Gage (1932) who worked with sinusoidal tones, and Harris (1960) who worked with filtered clicks. Considerable interest was given to this topic initially because of the hope that, since the latency of neural response was lower for sounds at higher intensity, there might be a single system based on interaural time differences responsible for lateralization. Thus, once acoustic intensity differences were translated to neural time differences, intensity might drop out as a separate factor, leaving lateralization based almost entirely upon interaural time differences.

However, subsequent studies by Whitworth and Jeffress (1961), Hafter and Jeffress (1968), and Hafter and Carrier (1972) have shown that separate images—one based on time and one based on intensity—may be perceived by listeners with sufficient training. It should be kept in mind that headphone-induced opposition of intensity and temporal cues is not found in nature, so that considerable experience was needed with these novel relations before separation of intensity from temporal contributions could be achieved by listeners. It would seem that experiments on time-intensity trading require an optimal amount of training—with too little, the necessary discriminations cannot be made; with too much, independent images are perceived for time and intensity. Even with optimal training, there is considerable variability among subjects concerning the relative importance given to time and intensity.

SOME CAUTIONS CONCERNING INTERPRETATION OF STUDIES USING HEADPHONES

Headphone experiments differ from normal listening conditions in important respects. With headphones, even when cues such as time and intensity are not deliberately placed in an anomalous relation (as in experiments with time-intensity trading), stimuli are abnormal and usually appear to have a source located within the listener's skull rather than out in the environment. When listening to external sources, extensive complex changes in the acoustic stimulus reaching the eardrums are produced by room acoustics, head shadows, pinnae reflections, and interaction of the sound with the neck and torso. The nature of these changes varies with the listener's distance and orientation relative to the source. While it might be thought at first that perceptual interpretation would be simpler and more direct when these complex stimulus transformations are blocked, further consideration suggests that what appears to be of staggering complexity to an experimenter describing stimuli and their transformations corresponds to the norm which we have learned to deal with. Any change from this norm leads to unusual and conflicting information. Headphone sounds, especially when heard diotically without echoes, are in some ways more similar to self-generated sounds (e.g., our own voice, chewing sounds, coughing) localized within our head than they are to sounds with external origins. Hence, considerable caution must be used in applying results of experiments using headphones to localization of real sources in the environment, since *stabilizing and simplifying stimulus configurations may complicate and confuse perception.* Considering this rule in another way, complex covariance of stimulus attributes associated with positional changes of an external source may be required for clear positional images. The extremely complex transformations produced by the pinnae, and required for optimal accuracy in localization, illustrate this principle.

IMPORTANCE OF THE PINNA IN SOUND LOCALIZATION

Charles Darwin considered that the pinnae were of little value for sound localization in man, believing them to be vestigial remnants of more elaborate structures used for localizing sounds by other animals. However, Rayleigh (1907) considered that the pinnae permit us to distinguish between sounds originating in front and behind. Butler (1969) and Blauert (1969/70), among others, have provided evidence that the pinnae furnish information concerning the location of a source in the medial plane in terms of both front/back position and elevation. These pinna cues appear to be primarily monaural, so that interaural comparison is not essential.

Batteau (1967, 1968) proposed a theory concerned with the effect of echoes produced by the corrugations of the pinnae on the intensities of high frequency components (above 6,000 Hz). He considered that these echo-induced intensity transformations provided information concerning azimuth as well as the elevation and front/back position in the medial plane. His conclusions were based upon measurements using a model constructed from a cast of a human pinna, but enlarged to five times normal size. Microphones placed at the entrance of the ear canal of the model measured echo delays from various azimuth and elevation angles. After scaling down results to apply to the normal pinna, Batteau concluded that azimuth angles introduced delays from 2 to 80 μsec and elevation angles introduced delays from about 100 to 300 μsec, the delays being monotonic functions for both azimuth and elevation. Batteau then used casts of the listeners' pinnae mounted on a stand, with microphone inserts at the position of the ear canals (without a model of the head between the pinnae). He found that, when sounds picked up by the microphones were heard by the listener through headphones, it was possible to create an externalized auditory image with accurate azimuth and elevation relevant to the artificial pinnae. Removal of the pinnae leaving only the bare microphones on the supporting stand destroyed localization ability. Batteau claimed that pinna convolutions producing time delays are not a peculiarity of human hearing—similar convolutions were found at the base of the ears of all mammals he examined. While he also stated that all species of birds he looked at had hard acoustically reflecting feathers forming a "pinna-like structure" surrounding the ear canal, recent evidence indicates that birds may utilize rather different physical principles than mammals for localization. Birds have an air-filled interaural passage which could correspond to a pressure-difference sensing system based on the acoustic coupling of the two tympanic membranes (Lewis & Coles, 1980).

Freedman and Fisher (1968) continued Batteau's line of experimentation. They found that it was not necessary to use the listener's own pinnae for modifying the input to the pick-up microphones—casts of someone else's pinnae could enhance accuracy of localization to some extent. They also reported that only a single pinna was necessary for localization and, when the distance between the artificial pinnae was increased to double the normal interaural distance (confounding binaural time differences and pinna cues), some localization was still associated with the acoustic effects produced by the pinnae.

Wright, Hebrank, and Wilson (1974) noted that questions had been raised concerning the ability of listeners to detect the very short monaural time delays required by Batteau's theory (see Davis, 1968), and they attempted to test for this ability directly. They found that monaural delay times of 20 μsec were detected easily when the amplitude ratio of the delayed to the leading signal was greater than 0.67. A digital delay line was used to simulate the action of the pinna as shown in figure 2.8, and Wright and his colleagues attributed the detection of delays to acoustic interaction resulting in high frequency attenuation for delay times under 30 μsec, and to multiple spectral intensity notches for longer delays (see Fig. 2.9). It is important to emphasize that, when listening to external sources, these large spectral changes are not perceived as alterations in the quality of the stimulus, but rather in terms of an unchanging stimulus subjected to alteration in position.

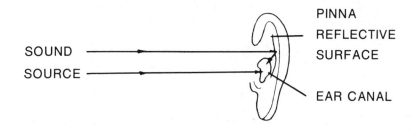

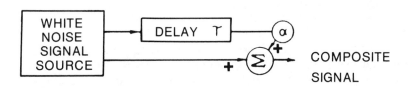

Fig. 2.8. Diagram of the generation of a time delay for a composite signal produced by pinna reflection, and the electronic circuit used in experiments simulating delays produced by the pinna.

Source: From D. Wright, J.H. Hebrank, and B. Wilson, "Pinna Reflections as Cues for Localization," *Journal of the Acoustical Society of America* 56 (1974): 957-62.

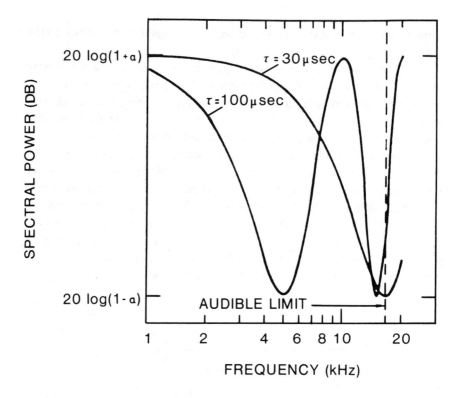

Fig. 2.9. Spectral filtering produced by combining a broad-band noise with a delay of itself. Delays less than 30 μsec cause low-pass filtering and delays greater than 30 μsec cause multiple spectral notches (α = ratio of delayed to undelayed signal amplitude; τ = time delay in μsec).
Source: From D. Wright, J.H. Hebrank, and B. Wilson, "Pinna Reflections as Cues for Localization," *Journal of the Acoustical Society of America* 56 (1974): 957-62.

There have been a few studies concerning the effect of changing or eliminating pinna interaction with sound upon the detection of elevation. Roffler and Butler (1968) had reported that, with normally positioned pinnae, listeners could identify with ease which source was radiating sound when two loudspeakers in the medial plane were separated in elevation by 11°. But performance in this task fell to chance level when they flattened and covered the pinnae using a plexiglass headband having an aperture over the opening of each ear canal. Gardner and Gardner (1973) studied the effect of occluding the cavities of the pinnae with plastic material on the ability to detect elevation in the medial plane. The accuracy of localization decreased with increased filling of the cavities, and no one portion of a pinna seemed more important than another.

ROOM ACOUSTICS

Plenge (1974) reasoned that listeners should not be able to localize sources within rooms unless they were familiar with both the nature of the sound and the acoustics of the room. He claimed that his subjects could achieve external localization of sounds delivered through headphones when the stimulus resembled a familiar sound in a familiar room; otherwise, the source appeared to be located within the head, as is usually the case when listening through headphones. Plenge stated that only a few seconds of listening was sufficient for calibration of a room's acoustic properties, which were stored as long as the listener remained in the room and then cleared immediately upon leaving, so that the listener could recalibrate at once for a new acoustic environment.

While Plenge has suggested that listeners can adjust very rapidly to the acoustics of a particular room, there is evidence that listeners also can adapt to (or compensate for) long-term changes in auditory cues.

AUDITORY REORIENTATION

There have been reports going back to the last century that accurate directional localization may be found in complete or partial monaural deafness, indicating that a recalibration of cues to localization had taken place. Conductive deafness is of special interest, since it is possible to compensate for, or to remove, the blockage and restore normal hearing. If the blockage is due to a plug of cerumen (wax) in the external ear canal, the procedure is especially simple and can be accomplished in a few minutes by syringing. Bezold (1890) reported that, when normal hearing was restored by removal of cerumen in one ear, there was a period of localization confusion lasting for a few weeks while readaption to "normal" hearing took place. Bergman (1957) described the consequences of operations on people with conductive hearing losses, and also stated that, along with an increase in acuity in one ear after the operation, there was a period of localization confusion which was not present before the operation.

Other experiments have reported that similar changes in localization could be produced experimentally by maintaining an artificial blockage in one ear for enough time to permit adjustment of localization to this condition, followed by removal of this blockage (for summary of this literature, see Jongkees & Veer, 1957).

In addition to these dramatic changes in localization criteria, there is a slow recalibration which we have all experienced. During childhood, the dimensions of head and pinna change, and our criteria for localization must change accordingly if accuracy is to be maintained.

There have been several experiments reported which have used "pseud-ophones" to alter localization cues. The first of these was by Thompson (1882) who was impressed both by Wheatstone's discovery of the stereo-scope and Wheatstone's construction of a "pseudoscope" in which binocular cues to distance were inverted by interchanging inputs to the right and left eyes. Thompson designed an instrument he called the "pseudophone" which had reflecting flaps for directing sounds into the ears from front, back, above, or below. The experimenter could manipulate the flaps on pseudophones worn by blindfolded subjects and so change the apparent position of sound sources. Young (1928) used a rather different type of a pseudophone consist-ing of two funnels mounted on the head which gathered sound that could be led to the ears through separate tubes. He studied the adaptation of localiza-tion to inversion produced by lateral cross-over of the sound-conducting tubes. Young's work was replicated and extended by Willey, Inglis, and Pearce (1937). These studies found that while listeners could learn to respond appropriately to side reversal of the ear trumpets, there was no complete auditory reorientation to pseudophones even after periods as long as a week. The lack of complete adaptation, perhaps, was not too surprising since the trumpets were quite different from pinnae, and the transformations produced were more than a simple lateral inversion of normal input.

Held (1955) used an electronic pseudophone, which consisted of hearing aid microphones mounted 20 cm apart on a bar attached to a headband worn by the subject. The bar formed an angle of 22° relative to the line joining the subject's ears, so that Held considered that he had shifted the interaural axis by 22°. The microphones were each used to power an ipsilateral earphone worn under a muff which attenuated normal airborne stimulation. Listeners wearing this device for a day could adapt appropriately and go through their normal daily activities without disorientation. But, at the end of the day, when the pseudophone was reset to produce no change from the anatomical interaural axis (setting of 0°), listeners reported two images, one correctly localized, and one displaced to the side opposite to that of the earlier axis shift produced by the pseudophone.

ESTIMATES OF DISTANCE FROM THE SOURCE

Near the turn of the century, a number of experiments demonstrated the ability of listeners to estimate distances of sources with considerable accu-racy (Matsumoto, 1897; Shutt, 1898; Starch & Crawford, 1909). Other studies have shown that there is "loudness constancy" or "loudness invariance" by which listeners can compensate for changes produced by varying the distance of the listener from the source (Fieandt, 1951; Mohrmann, 1939; Shigenaga, 1965). Let us consider the cues used by listeners in estimating the distance of a sound source.

Perhaps the most obvious cue to an increase in distance is a decrease in intensity. As a reasonably close approximation, the intensity (power) of a sound reaching the listener directly from the source is inversely proportional to the square of the distance (the inverse square law), so that a two fold change in distance corresponds to a four fold (6 dB) change in intensity. It has been recognized for a long time that intensity is a major cue to the distance of familiar sounds (see Pierce, 1901; Thompson, 1882). However, intensity is not the only cue to distance of a source: the ratio of direct to reverberant sound can be another important cue under some conditions.

If estimates of attenuation corresponding to a particular distance change (say doubling distance) are obtained in an experiment in which other cues normally changing with distance are held constant, a conflict of intensity reduction (indicating an increased distance) with other unchanging cues (indicating a fixed distance) can produce errors in estimating the relation between intensity and distance. If, on the other hand, all cues to distance covary in an experiment (as they would in the listener's experience outside the laboratory), then it is not possible to separate the contributions made by each of the possible cues. However, there does appear to be a way of avoiding this dilemma, which permits a direct determination of whether subjects can estimate the manner in which intensity changes with distance without other cues, either concordant or conflicting, to acoustic perspective. This may be accomplished by having the subjects generate the sounds themselves.

In an experiment dealing with the ability to estimate the attenuation of self-generated sounds with distance, subjects produced the vowel "ah," the unvoiced consonant "sh," and a pitchpipe tone (Warren, 1968a). These sounds were chosen so that they would be generated through the action of different physical principles and different muscular efforts. Subjects were requested to compensate for the effect of doubling distance to a target microphone. The instructions directed them first to produce one of the sounds at a comfortable level when the microphone was 10 feet away, and next to change the level of the sound so that it would remain unchanged at the position of the pick-up microphone when its distance was decreased to 5 feet. (The microphone was in view for both distances.) It was found that subjects (introductory psychology students) with no prior experience in auditory experiments or special knowledge of acoustic theory could compensate quite accurately for the effect of changing distance upon intensity, decreasing the intensities of their production by values close to the theoretical value of 6 dB.

As mentioned earlier, there is evidence that, when listeners are functioning as receivers rather than generators of sound, reverberation may function as an important cue to distance. When listening to external sources in rooms with normal characteristics, the ratio of direct to reverberant sound decreases with distance. In an experiment by Steinberg and Snow (1934), a person who was speaking at a fixed intensity moved back from a pick-up microphone while the gain was changed by the experimenter, so that the amplitude delivered to the listener through loudspeakers remained fixed. Under these conditions, the talker seemed to recede from the listener, an effect attributed by Steinberg and Snow to a change in the proportion of reverberant sound. Békésy (1938) reported similar results when he used equipment designed to change the ratio of direct to reverberant sound while keeping the overall amplitude fixed. In recent years, Mershon and King (1975) and Butler, Levy, and Neff (1980) reported that noise generated under reverberant conditions seemed much further away than noise generated in an anechoic room.

Maxfield (1930, 1931) described the importance of matching what he called "acoustic perspective" to visual perspective in making sound movies. It was pointed out that since binaural suppression of echoes (which will be discussed shortly) was not possible with one channel recordings, the overall level of reverberation must be decreased below the normal level to appear normal. He found it necessary to vary the proportion of direct to reverberant sound by appropriate positioning of the microphone when the camera position was changed in order to maintain realism. Maxfield gave an example of a long-shot sound track used with a close-camera shot which made it seem that the actors' voices were coming through an open window located behind them, rather than from their lips. He also made the very interesting observation that correct matching of acoustic and visual perspective influenced intelligibility: when a long-shot picture was seen, a long-shot sound track was more intelligible than a close-up sound track despite the fact that the increased reverberation would make it less intelligible if heard alone.

The delayed versions of a sound produced by echoes not only give rise to an acoustic perspective, but can also impart a pleasing "lively" character to voice and music (as opposed to an undesirable so-called "dead" quality when echoes are much reduced). The ability to minimize interference of masking by echoes has been rediscovered many times, and it goes by a number of names including "precedence effect," "Haas effect," "law of the first wave-front," and "first arrival effect" (see Gardner, 1968, for review). While reduction of masking caused by echoes works best with binaural listening, there is a considerable echo-suppression effect even without binaural differences. I have found that it is possible to demonstrate this single channel suppression effect for speech by comparing a recording with a low normal reverberation with one which was identical, except that the reverberant sound preceded the direct sound. The reversed reverberation recording was derived from a master tape prepared in an acoustically dead studio with the microphone a few inches from the talker's mouth. This tape was played in a reversed direction into a room having normal reverberation characteristics. An omni-directional pick-up microphone used for rerecording the speech was placed within two feet of the loudspeaker producing the reversed speech. When the backwards rerecording with the newly added reverberation was reversed once again on playback, the double reversal resulted in the speech being heard in the normal direction, but with reverberation preceding the voice. The slow build-up of reverberation preceding the sounds of speech and the abrupt drop in intensity at silent pauses seemed quite bizarre and was extremely noticeable. However, a rerecording prepared from the same mas-ter tape in a fashion which was identical, except that the reverberation was added in the normal temporal direction, resulted in a speech signal having a barely detectable reverberant quality. It appeared as if reverberation in the normal direction was incorporated within the speech, being transformed to a natural-sounding "lively" quality.

Gardner (1969) tested the ability of listeners to estimate distance from the source of a voice in a large anechoic room at the Bell Telephone Laborato-ries. Echoes were effectively abolished by the use of wedges of appropriate composition and shape placed along the walls, ceiling, and floor. Listeners and equipment were suspended between floor and ceiling on a wire-mesh support which did not reflect sound appreciably. When a voice was recorded and played back over loudspeakers at distances varying from 3 to 30 feet, estimates were independent of actual distance. However, when a "live" voice was used, an accuracy better than chance in estimating actual distances was found, especially for distances of a few feet. Gardner speculated that the ability of the listener to estimate distance when close to the talker could have resulted from audibility of nonvocal breathing, acoustic cues to the degree of effort made in producing the level heard, detection of echoes from the talker's body during conversational interchanges, radiation of body heat, and olfac-tory cues. Incidentally, the acoustic cues of vocal effort are not necessary concomitants of changes in vocal level. Talley (1937) stated that stage actors are capable of producing a special "audience speech" in which the fact that two people separated by a few feet are conversing at the level of a shout can be disguised by appropriate control of voice quality, so that the illusion is produced that they are communicating with each other rather than with the audience.

Mershon and his associates (Mershon & Bowers, 1979; Mershon & King, 1975), as the result of experiments with bursts of broad-band noise in both anechoic and ordinary rooms, concluded that, while intensity func-tioned as a cue to relative distance, reverberation could function as an absolute cue even when listeners had very little experience relating to the acoustic properties of the room. However, as mentioned earlier, Plenge (1974) has suggested that very little time and information is needed for listeners to determine the acoustic properties of rooms.

There is another cue to distance which comes into play out-of-doors at relatively great distances. Helmholtz (1877) noted that consonants with their high frequencies did not carry very far, stating that "It is interesting in calm weather to listen to the voices of the men who are descending from high hills to the plain. Words can no longer be recognized, or at most only such as are composed of M, N, and vowels as *Mamma, No.* But the vowels contained in the spoken word are easily distinguished. They form a strange series of alternations of quality and singular inflections of tone, wanting the thread which connects them into words and sentences." In keeping with this observation, Bloch (1893), after experiments with a variety of stimuli, concluded that sounds lacking high frequency components sounded farther away than sounds containing high frequencies. Also, Levy and Butler (1978) and Butler, Levy, and Neff (1980) reported that low-pass noise appeared farther away than high-pass noise. Coleman (1963) presented values for the absorption coefficient in dB/100 ft. for different frequencies, which showed that higher frequencies are attenuated much more than lower. He noted that this attenuation was highly dependent upon water-vapor content of the air. The calculations he presented show that at "typical conditions" encountered in a temperate climate, components at 8,000 Hz may have an attenuation 3 dB greater than components at 1,000 Hz for each 100 feet of travel.

Békésy (1960) has claimed that there are cues to apparent distance resulting from the spherical shape of wavefronts corresponding to sources within a few feet from listeners. At these short distances, an increase in low frequency components seems to make the source appear closer to the listener—a result in the opposite direction to that obtained with sounds coming from distant sources (which have wavefronts which can be considered as flat rather than curved).

SENSORY INPUT AND PHYSICAL CORRELATES

We have seen that changes in the nature of sensory input caused by shifts in the location of a source are perceived in terms of positional correlates, not in terms of the sensory changes themselves. As Helmholtz has stated "...we are exceedingly well trained in finding out by our sensations the objective nature of the objects around us, but...we are completely unskilled in observing the sensations *per se.* ..." (see Warren & Warren, 1968, p. 179). In chapter 4, evidence will be discussed indicating that, when attempts are made to have subjects estimate sensory magnitudes directly by judging relative subjective intensity (loudness) of sounds, responses are obtained which are based upon physical correlates associated with auditory localization.

3

Perception of Acoustic Repetition: Pitch and Infrapitch

This chapter reviews a classical problem, perception of tones, and suggests that our understanding of this topic may be enhanced by considering it as part of a larger topic: that of perception of acoustic repetition. As we shall see, periodic sounds repeated at tonal and infratonal frequencies appear to form a single perceptual continuum, with study in one range enhancing understanding in the other.

TERMINOLOGY

Some terms used in psychoacoustics are ambiguous. The American National Standards Institute has published a booklet on Psychoacoustical Terminology (ANSI S3.20-1973) which defines some basic technical words as having two meanings, one applying to the stimulus and the other to the sensation produced by the stimulus. The confusion of terms describing stimuli and their sensory correlates is an old one, and a potential cause of conceptual confusions—a danger that in 1730 led Newton (1952, p. 124) to warn that it is incorrect to use such terms as red light or yellow light, since "...the Rays to speak properly are not coloured." However, the ANSI definitions for the term *tone* reflect current usage, and state that the word can refer either to: (1) a sound wave capable of exciting an auditory sensation having pitch; or (2) a sound sensation having pitch. A similar ambiguity involving use of the same term to denote both stimulus and sensation is stated formally in the ANSI definitions for the word *sound*. The use of both of these terms will be restricted here to describe only the stimuli. The term *pitch* is defined as the attribute of auditory sensation which can be ordered on a scale extending from high to low.

The ANSI recommendation considers that the pitch of any particular sound can be described in terms of the frequency of a sinusoidal tone judged to have the same pitch, so that pitch is limited to the audible frequency range of sinusoidal tones extending from about 20 through 16,000 Hz. However, acoustic repetition can be perceived at rates well below the pitch limit for waveforms other than sinusoids, and we will name such sounds with detectable repetition as *infratones* or infratonal stimuli and their corresponding sensory attribute as *infrapitch*. Thus, the topic of detectable acoustic repetition involves both tonal and infratonal sounds producing sensations of pitch and infrapitch, respectively. The term *iterance* will be used as a general term encompassing the perceptual attributes of both pitch and infrapitch.

PITCH

The ancient Greeks appreciated that sounds correspond to vibratory movement of the air, and analogies were made between sound vibrations and water waves (see Hunt, 1978). They had an interest in the nature of pitch and the basis for musical intervals, and Pythagoras in the sixth century B.C. noted that simple integral ratios of the length of two vibrating strings corresponded to the common intervals (i.e., a ratio of 2:1 for an octave, a ratio of 3:2 for a fifth). In the seventeenth century, Galileo noted that if the Greeks had varied the pitches produced by a string by altering either the diameter or the tension rather than length, then pitch would have been found proportional to the square root of the physical dimension, and the octave and fifth would correspond to ratios of 4:1, and 9:4 respectively. Galileo then described an elegant experiment demonstrating that the octave did indeed correspond to a frequency ratio of 2:1. He observed that when the rim of a goblet containing water was stroked, standing waves appeared on the surface of the liquid. By slight changes in the manner of stroking it was possible to have the pitch jump an octave and, when that occurred, the standing waves changed in length by a factor of precisely two. Galileo also noted that, when a hard metal point was drawn over the surface of a soft brass plate, a particular pitch could be heard while, at the same time, a series of grooves with a periodic pattern appeared on the brass surface. When the spacing of two sets of periodic patterns corresponding to the musical interval of a fifth were compared, they were found to have the ratio of 3:2, indicating that this was the ratio of acoustic periodicities producing this interval.

Modern experimental work on pitch perception may be considered to have started with Seebeck's experiments with a siren (see Fig. 3.1). By forcing puffs of compressed air through holes in a rotating disc, periodic sounds consisting of a variety of puff-patterns were produced corresponding to the choice of distances separating the holes. For example, when the disc contained holes separated by the distances a, then b, then a, etc. (a, b, a, b, a, ...), the pitch heard was equivalent to that produced by a disc containing half the number of holes with a single distance c (equal to a + b) separating adjacent openings. When the distances a and b were made equal, the apparent period was halved, and the pitch increased by one octave. Seebeck (1841) concluded as a result of these experiments with repeated patterns consisting of two puffs, as well as more complex patterns, that the pitches heard corresponded to the period of the overall repeated pattern. Thus, it appeared to him that the number of complete statements of the periodic waveform per second

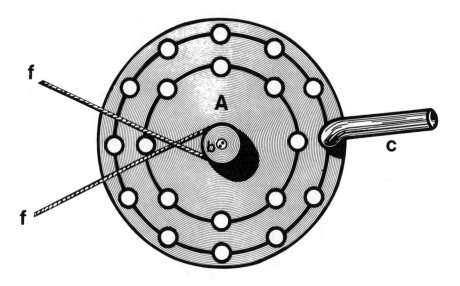

Fig. 3.1. The acoustic siren as used in Seebeck's time. Compressed air passing through tube (c) releases puff of air each time it is aligned with a hole in disk (A) which is rotated by cord (f) passing over a grooved driveshaft (b).
Source: From H.L.F. Helmholtz, *On the Sensations of Tone as a Physiological Basis for the Theory of Music* (New York: Dover, 1954).

determined the pitch. Ohm (1843) stated that Seebeck's contention that the pitches heard were based upon the repetition period of the overall pattern of puffs was incorrect, and that a Fourier analysis of the periodic signals into harmonic components took place with the pitch being determined by the frequency of the spectral fundamental. Seebeck (1843) countered by claiming that the spectral fundamental was not necessary for hearing a pitch equivalent to that frequency; he pointed out that, even when a spectral analysis showed that the fundamental was very weak or absent, the pitch of the fundamental (which corresponded to the waveform repetition frequency) was still the dominant pitch heard. The spectra of some of the stimuli generated by Seebeck as summarized by Schouten (1940a) are illustrated in figure 3.2. Seebeck suggested that the higher harmonic components might combine to cause the pitch corresponding to the fundamental to be heard, even when the fundamental was absent. As Schouten (1970) pointed out, this suggestion concerning the role of upper harmonics foreshadowed later non-

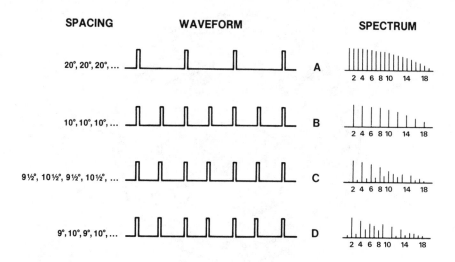

Fig. 3.2. Seebeck's waveforms and their corresponding spectra. The spacing of the holes in the siren's disk producing these sounds is given in degrees. The numbers used to describe the harmonics of the line spectra are based upon a waveform period corresponding to 20° (shown above as A).
Source: Adapted from J.F. Schouten, "The Residue, a New Component in Subjective Sound Analysis," *K. Acadamie van Wetenschappen, Amsterdam. Afdeeling Natuurkunde* (Proceedings) 43 (1940): 356-65.

spectral theories (including his own). Ohm (1844) had dismissed Seebeck's observations that a pitch could be heard corresponding to an absent or weak fundamental as merely an auditory illusion, to which Seebeck (1844) replied that the term "illusion" was inappropriate since only the ear could decide how tones should be heard. [For review of this controversy between Seebeck and Ohm see Schouten (1970) and de Boer (1976).] In the second half of the nineteenth century, Helmholtz (1877) backed Ohm's position in this controversy. Considering the ear an imperfect spectral analyzer, Helmholtz described distortion products which were capable of generating the fundamental frequency within the ear, even when missing as a Fourier component of a periodic stimulus. Helmholtz was well aware that a complex tone appears to have a single pitch rather than a cluster of pitches corresponding to the individual harmonics, and he attributed the perception of a single pitch to the adoption by unskilled listeners of a "synthetic" mode of listening to the entire complex of components, rather than an "analytical" mode in which component harmonics could be abstracted. Helmholtz stated that unskilled listeners could be trained to hear individual harmonics in a complex tone "with comparative ease." One recommended procedure involved first playing the harmonic component by itself at a soft level, and then immediately substituting the complex tone at a louder level: the harmonic could then be heard to continue as a component within the complex tone.

Helmholtz's position that sinusoidal components were responsible for the pitch of complex tones had great influence, largely because he offered a plausible explanation of how spectral analysis could be accomplished by the ear. As described in chapter 1, he suggested that the cochlea acted as if it contained a set of graded resonators each of which responded selectively to a particular component frequency. Low frequencies were considered to produce sympathetic vibrations at the apical end, and high frequencies at the basal end of the cochlea. His first version of the theory identified the rods of Corti as the resonant bodies, but this was later amended to consider resonating transverse fibers embedded in the basilar membrane as being responsible for spectral analysis. We have seen that Békésy modified the basis of Helmholtz's place theory from resonance to a traveling wave, with spectral analysis corresponding to the loci of maximal displacements produced by slow velocity waves (much slower than sound waves) sweeping along the basilar membrane from base to apex (see chapter 1). As discussed earlier, recent evidence indicates that spectral analysis may involve not only the loci of maximal displacements along the basilar membrane, but that the stereocilia of the receptor cells may perform a spectral analysis through resonant tuning (in a manner reminiscent of Helmholtz's original resonance theory involving the rods of Corti). The combination of basilar membrane movement and stereocilia resonance might provide a Fourier analysis of sounds at the level of receptor cells with finer sensitivity and spectral resolution than either mechanism operating alone.

There appears to be general agreement today that sound is subject to nonlinear distortions within the ear as Helmholtz had suggested. These distortions can introduce harmonic components when the stimulus consists of a sinusoidal tone, and can produce "combination tones" through the interaction of pairs of component frequencies. Among the more thoroughly studied combination tones are the simple difference tone ($f_2 - f_1$), and the cubic difference tone $(2f_1 - f_2)$. Thus, sinusoidal tones of 900 Hz and 1,100 Hz can produce a simple difference tone of 200 Hz and a cubic difference tone of 700 Hz.

While Helmholtz attributed the production of nonlinear distortion to the movements of the tympanic membrane and the ossicular chain within the middle ear, recent evidence has emphasized nonlinearity within the inner ear. However, there is no general agreement concerning the processes responsible for this nonlinearity (for reviews, see Green, 1976; Plomp, 1976).

Nonlinear distortions and the spectral analyses leading to pitch perception occur within the ear prior to neural stimulation. In addition, a temporal analysis of recurrent patterns of neural response appears to be involved in the perception of pitch. Before dealing with the temporal analysis of acoustic repetition, let us consider the topics of masking and critical bands which can help in understanding the nature of both frequency (place) and temporal (periodicity) coding.

Masking

It is well known that a louder sound can, under some conditions, mask (or prevent us from hearing) an otherwise audible fainter sound. Masking is not only a topic of direct practical interest, but also has been used widely to further our understanding of auditory processing.

Wegel and Lane (1924) used pure tones ranging from 200 Hz through 3,500 Hz as maskers. The masker was presented at a fixed SPL, and the threshold for a second sinusoidal (masked) tone was determined for various frequencies. Figure 3.3 presents their masked threshold function (sometimes called a masked audiogram) for different frequencies with a 1,200 Hz masker at 80 dB SPL. It can be observed that higher thresholds (corresponding to greater masking) were obtained for frequencies which were above rather than below the masking tone. The masked audiogram for frequencies near and above the frequency of the masker is marked by discontinuities or notches. There is general agreement on the basis for the notch centered on the masker frequency of 1,200 Hz: when two tones close to each other in frequency are mixed, a single pitch of intermediate frequency is heard, and the loudness fluctuations of first-order beats are heard. The beat rate is equal to the difference in frequencies of the tones, so that if the tones are 1,200 Hz and 1,206 Hz, beats are heard at the rate of six per second, with loudness minima occurring when the pressure crests of one sinusoidal waveform coincide with pressure troughs of the other. Thresholds of tones near the frequency of a masker are determined by just noticeable differences (jnd's) in intensity, and have been used to measure jnd's by Reisz (1928). The basis for the occurrence of notches at harmonics of the masker frequency is somewhat more controversial. Wegel and Lane attributed these dips to fluctuations in the intensity of the masked tone caused by interactions with aural harmonics of the masker (that is, harmonic distortion products generated within the ear), and these notches in the masking function have been used to estimate the extent of harmonic distortion (Fletcher, 1930; Lawrence & Yantis, 1956; Opheim & Flottorp, 1955). However, this explanation has been criticized on a variety of grounds (see Chocholle & Legouix, 1957a, 1957b; Meyer, 1957). Plomp (1967) studied the perceptual interaction of tones mistuned slightly from consonance, and provided evidence suggesting that higher order beats (that is, beats involving mistuning from consonance other than unison) are based upon detection of periodic fluctuations in the phase relations of the spectral components, even when these components are separated by several octaves. This comparison of temporal or phase information from widely separated cochlear loci could be responsible for the notches at harmonics of the lower frequency tone (2,400 Hz and 3,600 Hz) in figure 3.3.

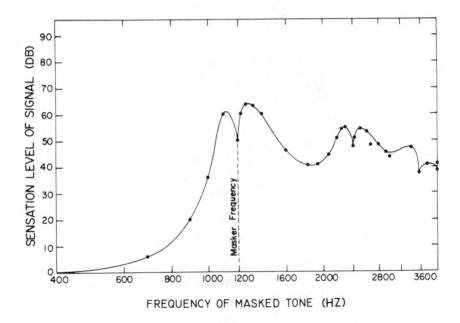

Fig. 3.3. Masking of one tone by another. The 1,200 Hz masker has a fixed intensity (80 dB SPL), and the masked threshold is given as sensation level (or dB above unmasked threshold).
Source: Adapted from R.L. Wegel and C.E. Lane, "The Auditory Masking of One Pure Tone by Another and its Probable Relation to the Dynamics of the Inner Ear," *Physical Review* 23 (1924): 266-85.

The complicating effects of beats in masking experiments can be reduced by using narrow-band noise as the masker. Figure 3.4 shows masked audiograms measured by Egan and Hake (1950) using a narrow-band noise centered at 410 Hz which was presented at various intensity levels. The notches observed with tonal maskers, if present at all, are very much reduced in magnitude, and the tonal threshold curves are almost symmetrical about the center frequency of the band of masking noise when it is present at its

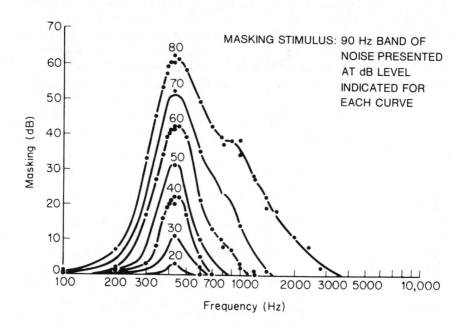

Fig. 3.4. Masking of tones by different levels of a narrow-band noise centered at 410 Hz.
Source: Adapted from J.P. Egan and H.W. Hake, "On the Masking Pattern of a Simple Auditory Stimulus," *Journal of the Acoustical Society of America* 20 (1950): 622-30.

lowest intensity levels. An upward spread of masking becomes quite pronounced at the highest intensity level: it can be seen in figure 3.4 that the threshold for a 1,500 Hz sinusoid is almost unaffected by a 70 dB narrow-band noise centered at 410 Hz, but a 10 dB increase in noise level raises the tonal threshold by more than 15 dB.

In addition to simultaneous masking, there are two types of nonsimultaneous masking. In "forward" masking, a louder preceding sound prevents detection of a brief faint sound. In "backward" masking, a brief faint sound is made inaudible by a louder subsequent sound. Both types of nonsimultaneous masking usually have effective durations of less than 100 msec.

Forward masking may correspond in part to the time required for the receptors to regain their sensitivity after exposure to a louder sound. This time is quite short, usually only tens of msec. Backward masking is more difficult to account for. One possible basis which has been suggested is that the subsequent louder sound produces neural activity which travels at a greater velocity and overtakes the fainter stimulus on the way to the central nervous system (Miller, 1947), thus effectively becoming a special case of simultaneous masking. Both forward and backward masking are frequency dependent, in a manner resembling that already described for simultaneous masking. (For further discussion, see Elliot, 1971.)

We are often surrounded by competing sounds which can interfere with signals of interest and importance through simultaneous masking, backward masking, and forward masking. However, signals do not always disappear when masked. This topic will not be pursued further now, but in chapter 6 we will discuss the rather sophisticated perceptual mechanisms capable of reversing the effects of masking and restoring acoustically obliterated signals.

Critical Bands

Fletcher (1940) interpreted earlier studies of masking as indicating that the basilar membrane operates as a filter having a limited resolving power corresponding to what he called a "critical band." He considered that louder sounds could prevent detection of (or mask) fainter sounds when they stimulated the same critical bands. Fletcher attempted to measure widths of critical bands at various center frequencies by using noise to mask tonal signals. The average power in a 1 Hz wide band within a broad-band noise is called the "noise power density" and abbreviated as N_0. Fletcher started with broad-band noise having a constant N_0 at all frequencies (that is, white or Gaussian noise), and measured the masked threshold for a tone presented along with the noise. He decreased the bandwidth of the noise keeping N_0 of the remaining noise fixed, and found that little or no effect was observed on the masked threshold when the frequencies removed from the noise were beyond a critical distance from the tone. Fletcher's conclusion that a narrow "critical band" is mainly responsible for masking is now generally accepted, and has proved extremely valuable in understanding the interaction of components having different frequencies. However, Fletcher made the further assumption that the total power of a noise within a critical band is the same as the power of a tone centered within that band at its masked threshold. This assumption has been questioned by Scharf (1970), who suggested that estimates of the width of the critical band based on the ratio of tonal power at masked threshold to N_0 are roughly 40 percent less than the width of the critical band measured by other methods involving direct frequency interactions on the basilar membrane. Values obtained using Fletcher's method are sometimes called "critical ratios," with the term "critical band" being reserved for values obtained with other procedures as shown in figure 3.5. However, Spiegel (1981) has argued recently that Fletcher's method is valid when used with suitable precautions, either for pure tones masked with noise of various bandwidths, or for narrow-band noise masked with wider-band noise.

Each critical band covers about the same distance on the basilar membrane, and Greenwood (1961) has estimated the width corresponding to a critical band to be approximately one millimeter.

Place Theory

De Boer (1976) and Moore (1977) both have pointed out that there are two place theories: one considers that there is a Fourier analysis of limited resolution along the basilar membrane, with lower frequencies stimulating the apical end and higher frequencies the basal end; the other considers that pitch is determined by the places stimulated. The first place theory is supported by overwhelming evidence; the second seems to be only partly true—that is, place is not the sole determinant of pitch. For a sinusoidal tone, the locus of maximum stimulation changes regularly with frequency only from about 50 through 16,000 Hz, so that place cannot account for low pitches from 20 through 50 Hz. Further, the just noticeable difference (jnd) in frequency of sinusoidal tones appears to be too small to be accounted for by spectral resolution along the basilar membrane. Figure 3.5 shows that for 500 Hz the critical band width is about 100 Hz, yet jnd's having values less than 1 Hz have been reported (Moore, 1974; Nordmark, 1968). While there are mechanisms based on place which have been proposed for discriminating tones separated by considerably less than a critical band (Békésy, 1960; Tonndorf, 1970; Zwicker, 1970), none seems capable of handling jnd's as small as those reported by Nordmark and by Moore.

A number of difficulties have been encountered by classical place theorists in dealing with the pitch of complex tones. As we have seen, a single pitch corresponding to the spectral fundamental is generally heard despite the presence of harmonic components stimulating regions associated with other pitches, and the fundamental frequency still characterizes the pitch of a complex tone even when it is not present as a component of the stimulus. Helmholtz (1877) described the generation of difference tones (that is, creation of frequencies corresponding to the difference between sinusoidal components) which could account for perception of the absent fundamental

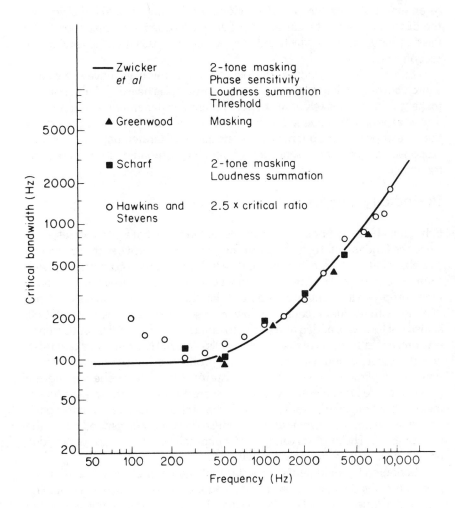

Fig. 3.5. The width of critical bands as a function of center frequency. Values are presented from several sources. Data of Hawkins and Stevens were transformed by multiplying their values (considered as "critical ratios") by 2.5.

Source: From B. Scharf, "Critical Bands," in J.V. Tobias (Ed.), *Foundations of Modern Auditory Theory.* Vol. 1 (New York: Academic Press, 1970), pp. 157-202.

(although Helmholtz does not seem to have used difference tones explicitly as an explanation of this problem). However, Fletcher (1924) did claim that the distortion within the ear could produce a frequency corresponding to a missing fundamental—which thus would not be missing at the level of the receptor cells.

Experiments conducted after Fletcher made this claim have shown that a pitch corresponding to the missing fundamental is heard under conditions making it highly unlikely that the fundamental is generated within the ear. These experiments have led to the development of temporal or periodicity theories of pitch perception, which consider that iterated patterns of neural response can produce a sensation of pitch corresponding to the repetition frequency.

Periodicity Theory

Schouten (1938) demonstrated in an elegant fashion that a pitch corresponding to the fundamental of a complex tone was heard even when this frequency was absent at the level of the receptor cells. He prepared a complex tone with a fundamental of 200 Hz, and first removed the fundamental by the addition of the appropriate intensity of a second 200 Hz sinusoidal tone that was 180° out of phase with the fundamental. Following this acoustic cancellation, a 206 Hz sinusoidal tone was added as a probe to determine if the 200 Hz fundamental was present at the level of the receptor cells—if a 200 Hz tone were generated within the ear, it would interact with the probe to produce periodic fluctuations in amplitude (or beats) at the rate of 6 Hz. The probe verified the absence of the fundamental. Yet a pitch corresponding to the missing fundamental could be heard clearly, although the quality associated with this pitch was quite different from that of a sinusoidal tone corresponding to the fundamental. These observations led Schouten to his concept of "residue pitch" which will be discussed shortly.

Schouten's experiments, showing that the pitch of the missing fundamental is carried by higher harmonics, requires subjects skilled in matching the pitch of tones having different qualities. Licklider (1954) demonstrated the same basic phenomenon in a manner which did not require such skills. At a meeting of the Acoustical Society of America, he first let the audience hear a recognizable melody consisting of a sequence of complex tones lacking lower harmonics. In order to show that the melody was carried by the upper harmonics, he then added a band of low frequency noise of sufficient intensity to mask any distortion products: the melody could still be heard quite clearly. Subsequent quantitative studies also have used low frequency masking noise to ensure that the spectral fundamental did not contribute to the pitch produced by higher harmonics of complex tones (Patterson, 1969; Small & Campbell, 1961).

Schouten's Residue Pitch

In a number of experiments, Schouten (1938, 1939, 1940a) verified and extended Seebeck's suggestion that higher harmonics of pulse trains could combine to produce the pitch of an absent fundamental.

Schouten first tried using an acoustic siren to generate pulses (as did Seebeck), and found that, while he could hear the auditory phenomena described by Seebeck, there was much variability in the stimulus and some undesired noise was produced. Schouten designed an "optical" siren, in which rotating masks of different shapes determined the pattern of light reaching a photosensitive cell, which then controlled the waveform of a signal driving a loudspeaker. The optical siren could not only produce intact pulse trains, but construction of appropriate masks permitted deletion of desired lower harmonics. (Fine adjustments in the masks were made with the help of a wave analyzer that measured the strength of individual spectral components.) As the result of his experiments, Schouten (1970) came to the following conclusions:

(1) The ear follows Ohm's law for frequencies wider apart than, say, a full tone (12%). In a harmonic series from 8 to 10 lower harmonics can be perceived by the unaided ear.
(2) Higher harmonics are heard collectively as one subjective component (one percept) called the residue.
(3) The residue has a sharp timbre.
(4) The residue has a pitch equal to that of the fundamental tone. If both are present in one sound they can be distinguished by their timbre.

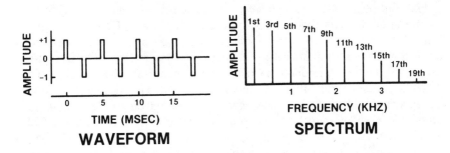

Fig. 3.6. Waveform and odd-harmonic spectrum of a 200 Hz alternating polarity pulse train. The harmonic number of each spectral line is numbered. Source: Adapted from J.F. Schouten, "The Residue, a New Component in Subjective Sound Analysis," *K. Akademie van Wetenschappen, Amsterdam. Afdeeling Natuurkunde* (Proceedings) 43 (1940): 356-65.

Schouten (1940a) realized that one possible objection to his explanation for residue pitch in terms of periodicity of the entire waveform could be that the difference between successive harmonics also is 200 Hz, and that this differ- ence might be responsible for the pitch of the residue. He produced a train of pulses of alternating polarity having a fundamental of 200 Hz (see Fig. 3.6). Any periodic sound consisting of waveforms alternating in polarity has a fundamental corresponding to the waveform repetition frequency, but lacks even numbered harmonics; hence, the spectral compositon of the alternating pulse trains was 200, 600, 1,000,.... Hz. Schouten stated that a residue pitch could be heard when listening to this stimulus without filtering, and that this pitch did not correspond to the difference frequency of 400 Hz, but to the waveform repetition frequency of 200 Hz. As we shall see, this choice of a 200 Hz stimulus was fortunate for his theory. Had he used a 100 Hz alternating polarity pulse train, he might have heard two simultaneous pitches of 100 Hz and 200 Hz with this interesting stimulus, and had he high-pass filtered his 200 Hz signal to remove the lower spectral components he might have heard a pitch of 400 Hz. We shall also see that perception of a frequency twice that of the fundamental, when it does occur, need not involve the perception of a difference tone.

Pitch of Inharmonic Complexes

Schouten (1940b) provided another demonstration indicating that residue pitch was not due to the perception of difference tones corresponding to the frequency separation of neighboring spectral components. He started with a complex tone having a frequency of 200 Hz (components at 200, 400, 600, ... Hz) and increased the frequency of each component by 40 Hz (240, 440, 640, ... Hz). Although the frequency difference between components was 200 Hz for the latter stimulus, this was not the pitch heard: the pitch changed slightly but reliably to a little more than 200 Hz. This type of pitch shift was later studied in a detailed quantitative manner by de Boer (1956). De Boer first presented the five component harmonic complex of 800, 1,000, 1,200, 1,400, 1,600 Hz, and observed that the fundamental of 200 Hz was heard as would be expected. When he increased each component by 50 Hz through an amplitude modulation technique to produce the complex of 850, 1,050, 1,250, 1,450, 1,650 Hz, the pitch heard was increased to about 210 Hz. De Boer offered an explanation for the pitch shift in terms of a central pitch extractor which constructed a harmonic complex most closely approximating the inharmonic complex. In the example given above, this would correspond to 833.3, 1,041.7, 1,250, 1,458.3, 1,666.7 Hz, with a missing fundamental of approximately 208.3 Hz (close to the experimentally found value). De Boer suggested that the pitch extractor employed place information for spectral components with low harmonic numbers which stimulated discrete loci and temporal information for those components with high harmonic numbers which could not be resolved by place of stimulation. He pointed out that, mathematically, these mechanisms (spectral and temporal) were equivalent.

Schouten, Ritsma, and Cardozo (1962) proposed a somewhat different model. They used amplitude modulated signals consisting of harmonically related components, such as 1,800, 2,000, 2,200 Hz, and then shifted the frequency of each component by the same amount to produce an inharmonic sequence. Pitch shifts similar to those reported by de Boer for his five component signals were observed. They also reported that while a harmonic three component complex such as that described above (1,800, 2,000, 2,200 Hz) had a dominant pitch corresponding to the amplitude modulation envelope (200 Hz), several fainter pitches could be heard as well (see Fig. 3.7). Schouten and his associates suggested a model in which the ambiguity was attributed to a pitch processor which measured time intervals between peaks as shown in the figure. They noted that increasing component frequencies by

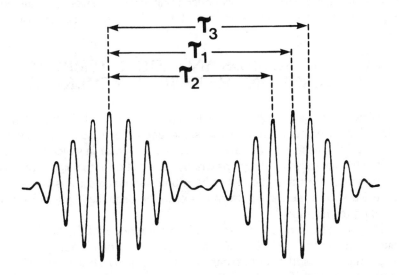

Fig. 3.7. Diagram describing behavior of a hypothetical pitch extractor which measures intervals between main peaks in a waveform. The waveform shown is that of a complex tone corresponding to the sinusoidal modulation of a carrier tone having a frequency ten times that of the modulation frequency. Some of the possible pitches are considered to be based on the intervals τ_1, τ_2, and τ_3.

Source: Adapted from J.F. Schouten, R.J. Ritsma, and B.L. Cardozo, "Pitch of the Residue," *Journal of the Acoustical Society of America* 34 (1962): 1418-24.

a fixed amount did not change the envelope repetition frequency of 200 Hz but did change the fine structure within the envelope. Since the pitch does change, they reasoned that fine structure must enter into pitch judgments. For further discussion of the topic of pitch shifts of inharmonic sequences of tones, see Plomp (1976).

Spectral Dominance

Since harmonic components of complex tones can generate a pitch matching that of the spectral fundamental, there have been attempts to determine which harmonics play the leading role in generating the pitch. Experiments by Ritsma (1962, 1963) suggested that components with low harmonic numbers play a dominant role. Subsequent experiments by Ritsma and by other investigators indicated that harmonic numbers from about three to five usually were the most important in establishing pitch (for reviews, see Plomp, 1976; Ritsma, 1970). While these dominant harmonics are resolvable along the basilar membrane, they also overlap in critical bands, so that both temporal and spatial information might be available for these components.

PERIODIC SOUNDS AND LOCAL TEMPORAL PATTERNS ON THE BASILAR MEMBRANE

In dealing with the possible bases for the residue pitch heard when all components were delivered to the same ear or ears, Schouten (1940c) considered the basilar membrane as a tuned resonator in which lower harmonics stimulated isolated regions without interaction with neighboring harmonics, while several of the higher harmonics stimulated the same region. Figure 3.8 shows the local pattern of excitation produced by a pulse train according to this model.

Plomp (1966) employed a more up-to-date model of the basilar membrane response to a 200 Hz pulse train, using a set of 1/3-octave filters to approximate the width of critical bands. Figure 3.9 shows tracings obtained in my laboratory using Plomp's method with pulses of 100 microseconds duration and 1/3-octave filters having attenuations of 30 dB one octave from the center frequencies of the filters. The tracings resemble closely those obtained by Plomp for the same stimulus. The responses of the filters, of course, still are not intended to represent the actual patterns along the basilar membrane in a quantitative fashion. However, the tracings do illustrate clearly some effects of the band-pass filtering occurring within the cochlea.

Both figures provide an impressive indication that bursts of activity having a periodicity corresponding to the pulse rate occur at cochlear loci which respond to frequencies several times higher than the spectral funda-

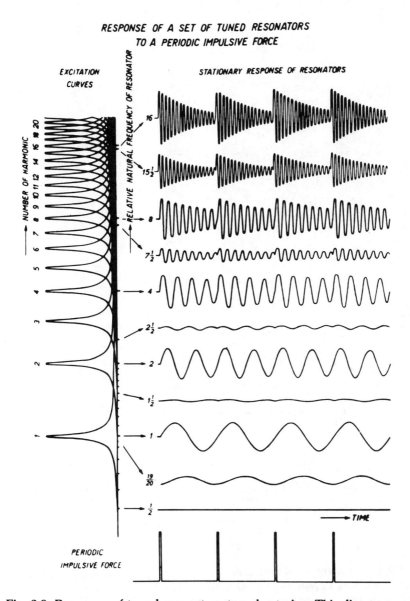

Fig. 3.8. Response of tuned resonators to pulse trains. This diagram represents a model of how cochlear resonators could permit both the spectral resolution of lower harmonics and the interaction of higher harmonics to produce periodic waveforms having maxima corresponding to the period of the pulse train.

Source: From J.F. Schouten, "The Residue and the Mechanism of Hearing," *K. Akadamie van Wetenschappen, Amsterdam. Afdeeling Natuurkunde* (Proceedings) 43 (1940): 991-99.

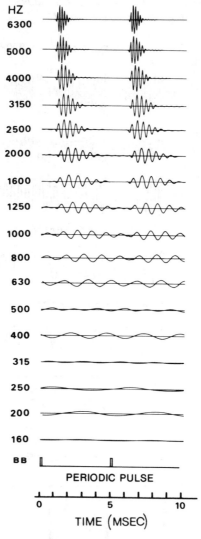

Fig. 3.9. Demonstration of the nature of the basilar membrane's response to pulse trains based upon Plomp's procedure (see text). Response curves are shown for a set of 1/3-octave filters having center frequencies of 160, 200, 250, ... 6,300 Hz stimulated simultaneously by a 200 Hz pulse train (shown diagramatically in broad-band form as BB at the bottom of the figure). Spectral resolutions of lower harmonics can be seen, as well as the emergence of pulsate patterns with repetition frequencies of 200 Hz for filters with the highest center frequencies. The same equipment and procedures was used in preparing the tracings for the nonpulsate stimuli shown in Figures 3.11, 3.13, and 3.18.

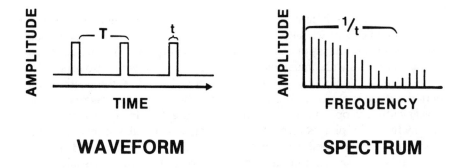

Fig. 3.10. Amplitude spectra of pulse trains. The spacing between spectral lines shown in the figure on the right equals 1/T Hz, where T is the period in seconds of the waveform shown on the left. The spectral harmonic with minimal amplitude is the one closest to 1/t Hz, where t is the pulse duration (or pulse width) in seconds.

mental. Detection of the burst frequency at these loci could lead to perception of residue pitch. However, pulse trains are rather special stimuli, and nonpulsate complex tones (which also exhibit residue pitch) do not produce such bursts of activity when filtered. In order to study general principles governing the perception of tones, it would seem desirable to use some model periodic stimulus lacking the special waveforms and spectra characteristic of specific types of sounds.

Let us turn for a moment to consideration of model and special stimuli in auditory research.

MODEL PERIODIC STIMULI
VERSUS SPECIAL PERIODIC STIMULI

Periodic stimuli of a particular frequency can have an almost limitless number of waveforms and spectra. One of the most important special stimuli is the simple or pure tone, since it consists only of a single spectral component. These sinusoidal waveforms have proved invaluable in studying cochlear mechanics, neural physiology, and pitch perception. However, pure tones are encountered infrequently outside the laboratory, and most of our experience with periodic sounds involves complex tones. Also, the thresholds for pure tones become so high below 20 Hz that they are effectively inaudible, while all other periodic waveforms can be heard at lower repetition frequencies.

In the nineteenth century, complex tones were generated by a siren or by a rotating Savart wheel (see Boring, 1942, p. 335), both of which could produce periodic pulses or clicks of any desired frequency. Today, electronic pulse generators with adjustable frequency and pulse width are used often when complex tones with broad spectra are desired. If the width of the periodic pulse is narrow, the amplitude of higher harmonics decreases only slowly with harmonic number, as shown in figure 3.10. However, the special alignment of the phases of spectral components of pulse trains produces unique patterns of auditory stimulation, as indicated in figures 3.8 and 3.9. Also, at low tonal and infratonal frequencies, pulse trains are unusual stimuli, sounding like a sequence of brief clicks separated by silence.

If we turn from pulses to familiar complex tones, such as the individual periodic sounds employed in speech and music, we find that they each have special qualities and a limited range of repetition frequencies. Is there, then, any sound which can be considered as a model periodic stimulus?

Iterated Noise Segments as Model Periodic Sounds

It has been suggested that iterated segments of Gaussian noise are useful as model stimuli for studying perception of periodic sounds (Warren & Bashford, 1981). Such stimuli have a randomly determined amplitude for individual spectral components and randomly determined relative phase relations among harmonic components. Thus, they can be considered as general cases of periodic stimuli with no *a priori* restrictions concerning the waveform, or the amplitude and phase spectra. As we shall see, it has been found that principles governing perception of randomly derived periodic waveforms apply to special waveforms as well. However, it should be noted that particular periodic sounds (such as vowels, sinusoidal tones, pulse trains, square waves, etc.) may have additional special rules superimposed upon more general ones.

Randomly derived periodic waveforms can be generated in a number of ways. In most of the studies described below, white or Gaussian noise was introduced into a digital delay line with the delay setting corresponding to the desired period. Upon switching the delay line to "recycle" mode, further input was rejected and the stored waveform repeated indefinitely in digital form. The digital to analog conversion resulted in "recycled Gaussian noise" or RGN. (For procedural details, see Warren & Bashford, 1978.) When, for example, the duration of the repeated noise segment is 5 msec, a complex tone is produced with a period of 5 msec and a frequency of 200 Hz. The pitch of the 200 Hz RGN is the same as that of a 200 Hz sinusoidal tone, but the timbre reflects the presence of higher harmonics. Every harmonic of 200 Hz within the audible range is present and, as mentioned earlier, each of the harmonics has a randomly determined amplitude and phase.

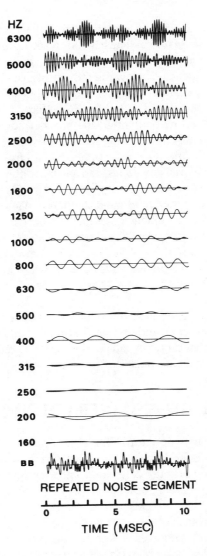

Fig. 3.11. Illustration of the nature of the basilar membrane response to a model periodic sound. Two statements of a repeated noise segment (period 5 msec, repetition frequency 200 Hz) are shown in unfiltered or broad-band form in the tracing labeled BB, with response curves obtained from the same set of 1/3-octave filters used for figure 3.9 shown directly above. The center frequencies of the filters are shown to the left of each response curve. Spectral resolution of the sinusoidal waveforms of the individual lower harmonics can be seen, as well as a series of iterated complex patterns (each with a period of 5 msec) produced by individual filters with center frequencies above 800 Hz. For additional details, see text.

It is of interest to compare the responses at different positions on the basilar membrane as simulated in figure 3.9 for a 200 Hz pulse train with the equivalent simulation shown in figure 3.11 for a 200 Hz RGN. For 1/3-octave bands with center frequencies below the fifth harmonic (1,000 Hz), there is evidence of spectral resolution of individual harmonics, and the response curves for the pulse trains (Fig. 3.9) and the RGN (Fig. 3.11) are quite similar. At center frequencies corresponding to the fifth harmonic and above, evidence of the interaction of neighboring harmonics within single 1/3-octave bands can be seen, and the response curves derived from pulse trains and RGNs differ. The waveform envelopes derived from pulse trains take on a characteristic pulsate structure, with synchronous bursts of activity corresponding to each pulse of the broad-band stimulus at each of the higher filter settings. There is no such resemblance of the 1/3-octave bands of the RGN either to each other or to the broad-band parent waveform. The waveforms of successive bands for the RGN above the fourth harmonic can be seen to have different randomly determined envelopes, usually with multiple maxima and minima. However, each of the 1/3-octave band waveforms has the same period of 5 msec.

The spectrally resolved lower harmonics are not required for hearing pitch. When the fundamental and first few harmonics of a 200 Hz RGN are removed by high-pass filtering, a clear "residue" pitch of 200 Hz can be heard resembling that obtained with pulse trains.

PITCH AND INFRAPITCH

Iterance can be heard with ease for RGNs over a range of 15 octaves, from about 0.5 Hz through 16,000 Hz. The perceptual characteristics for the entire continuum are depicted in figure 3.12 along with their possible neural bases. The boundaries for perceptual qualities and neural mechanisms are shown at discrete frequencies, but it should be kept in mind that these boundaries actually are gradual transitions occurring in the vicinity of the repetition frequencies indicated. Five octaves of detectable acoustic repetition lie within the infrapitch range (0.5 through 20 Hz). As we shall see, one of the mechanisms contributing to pitch appears to operate without the others at infrapitch frequencies.

When heard through standard laboratory headphones with a response limit of 8,000 Hz, RGNs above 4,000 Hz consist solely of the fundamental sinusoidal frequency (the second harmonic has a frequency above the 8,000 Hz response limit of the headphones), so that RGNs are indistinguishable from sinusoidal tones of the same repetition frequency. At repetition frequencies below about 2,000 Hz, RGNs take on a quality quite different from sinusoidal tones. Independent RGNs of the same frequency each have the

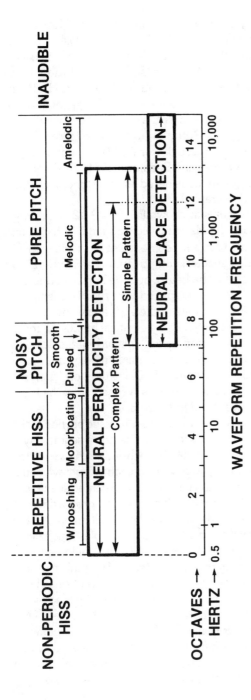

Fig. 3.12. Perception of acoustic repetition for model stimuli consisting of repeated segments derived from white noise. Waveform repetition frequency is designated in Hertz and also as the number of octaves above the lower limit of detectable iterance. The upper portion of the figure describes the perceptual characteristics; transitions between the qualities given are gradual, with category boundaries at the approximate positions shown. Possible neurological mechanisms for iterance at particular waveform frequencies are shown.

Source: Modified from R.M. Warren and J.A. Bashford, Jr., "Perception of Acoustic Iterance: Pitch and Infrapitch," *Perception & Psychophysics 29* (1981): 395-402.

same pitch but a different quality or timbre reflecting their individual wave-forms and spectra (Warren & Bashford, 1981). Warren and Bashford also reported that from about 100 through 20 Hz, RGNs have a pitch linked to a hiss-like quality. This noisy pitch seems continuous or smooth from about 100 through 70 Hz, and interrupted or pulsing from about 70 through 20 Hz. Pitch is absent for repetition frequencies below about 20 Hz. From roughly 20 through 4 Hz, iterated noise segments have a clear staccato sound which has been described as "motorboating" by Guttman and Julesz (1963). They described the perceptual quality from 4 through 1 or 0.5 Hz as "whooshing." In keeping with the suggestion of Warren and Bashford (1981), RGNs in the motorboating and whooshing ranges are considered as "infratones" produc-ing a detectable periodicity called "infrapitch."

Let us examine the neural mechanisms shown in figure 3.12 as subserv-ing detection of infratones. An RGN of 2 Hz can be considered as a harmonic sequence of sinusoidal components with a fundamental of 2 Hz and with a 2 Hz separation between neighboring spectral components. The lowest 25 or so harmonics lying below 50 Hz cannot be heard, and the higher harmonics which are in the audible range are too closely spaced to be resolved along the basilar membrane (see Plomp, 1964, for limits of the ear's analyzing power). Since many unresolved harmonics fall within a single critical band, and these interacting harmonics have randomly determined relative intensities and relative phases, highly complex local patterns of stimulation are produced at every stimulated locus on the basilar membrane. While the temporal patterns differ at separate loci, each of the complex patterns is repeated at the RGN repetition frequency of 2 Hz, as illustrated in figure 3.13.

This figure shows the patterns corresponding to a 10 msec portion of the 500 msec period of a 2 Hz iterated noise segment. The noise segment was excised from pink noise band-passed from 100 through 10,000 Hz. Since the long-term spectrum of pink noise has equal power for each 1/3-octave band, the patterns at the lower frequencies shown in figure 3.13 can be seen more clearly than they could be for white noise for which power is proportional to the center frequency of 1/3-octave bands. It should be kept in mind that the temporal patterns for the 2 Hz signal are quite long and complex, each being fifty times the 10 msec portion shown in the figure. Also, it should be noted that while not all audible 1/3-octave bands are depicted, comparable patterns repeated each 500 msec would be created for each such band. It has been demonstrated that information concerning infrapitch periodicity is available along the entire length of the basilar membrane, for when a 1/3-octave filter was swept through a broad-band infratonal RGN, the repetition frequency was heard at all center frequencies of the filter (Warren & Bashford, 1981). Identification of the 2 Hz repetition could be accomplished only through a temporal analysis of the iterated complex pattern of neural response.

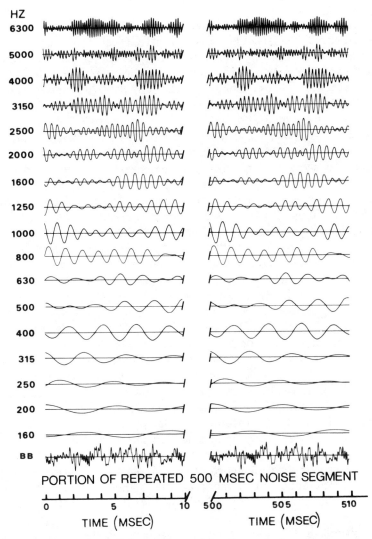

Fig. 3.13. Illustration of the nature of basilar membrane response to an iterated 500 msec segment of pink noise (repetition frequency, 2 Hz). Ten msec of the broad-band (BB) waveform is shown at the bottom of the figure, with output waveforms of the same set of 1/3-octave filters used for Figure 3.9 displayed above. The center frequency of each filter is shown at the left of its response curve. The last 490 msec of each waveform are not shown: the tracings in the figure recommence with the next restatement of the beginnings of the iterated patterns. As indicated by the tracings, each of the 1/3-octave filters generated a different complex pattern, with each pattern having the same repetition frequency of 2 Hz.

At acoustic repetition frequencies greater than about 50 to 100 Hz, the fundamental and the first few harmonics of an RGN can be resolved along the basilar membrane. These spatially resolved sinusoidal components produce the local excitation maxima providing the basis for the "neural place detection" cues to repetition frequency shown in figure 3.12. Nerve fibers originating at the places of excitation maxima receive stimulation at or near their characteristic frequency, and their firing exhibits phase-locking to the local frequency up to 4,000 or 5,000 Hz (see chapter 1). The interspike intervals associated with phase-locking can provide temporal information concerning frequency (as shown in Fig. 1.16). This temporal cue based on spectrally resolved harmonics is designated as "simple pattern" in figure 3.12 and, as indicated, can furnish information concerning RGN frequencies from a lower limit of about 50 or 100 Hz to an upper limit of about 4,000 to 5,000 Hz.

In addition to the phase-locked simple pattern, there is another class of temporal cues available for determining some frequencies of tonal RGNs. As illustrated in the simulation of the basilar membrane's response to a 200 Hz RGN in figure 3.11, when a nerve fiber's characteristic frequency is several times greater than the repetition frequency of an RGN, periodic "complex patterns" may modulate the responses of a fiber. This complex pattern period is the same as the RGN period (see Fig. 3.11). RGNs above a few kiloHertz do not produce complex pattern cues to repetition frequency since they do not have the unresolved upper harmonics necessary for generation of these patterns on the basilar membrane. The lower limit of the operating range for complex pattern cues to RGN frequency is about 0.5 Hz. As we have seen, at infratonal RGN frequencies, perception of iterance cannot be based upon either neural place or phase-locked simple pattern cues, and appears to be based solely upon detection of the repetition of complex patterns.

Let us summarize the types of neural information available for the perception of iterance with our model periodic stimuli. There are three types of cues, each functioning over a limited range of frequencies: (1) neural place information, requiring spectral resolution of lower harmonics, and operating from a lower limit of 50-100 Hz up to the frequency limit of hearing at about 16,000 Hz; (2) phase-locked simple pattern information operating from a lower limit of about 50-100 Hz through 4,000-5,000 Hz, which supplements place information carried by the same nerve fibers; and (3) complex pattern information operating for RGNs with frequencies from about 0.5 Hz through perhaps 2,000 Hz, which is carried by auditory nerve fibers having characteristic frequencies lying between a lower limit several times greater than the waveform repetition frequency up to the limit of audibility (about 16,000 Hz).

How can the repetition of complex patterns corresponding to infratonal RGNs (such as those illustrated in Fig. 3.13) be detected? Warren and Bashford (1981) presented evidence along several lines that, while exceptional features of temporal patterns at discrete loci on the basilar membrane might be detectable for repetition at infratonal frequencies, it appeared also that the overall temporal pattern of neural response was stored and recognized holistically when iterated. One line of evidence indicating a holistic pattern recognition involved splitting an infratonal RGN into three parts of equal duration which can be called A, B, and C. When reassembled to form the RGNs $(ABC)_n$ and $(ACB)_n$, these permuted orders were readily distinguished even by untrained listeners. Therefore, relations across items within the patterns were detectable. If only repetition of isolated exceptional features within A, B, and C were detected without cross-item integration, then the permuted orders should not have been distinguishable.

Perception of Multiple Infratonal Frequencies Stimulating the Same Cochlear Loci

Pairs of infratonal RGNs having repetition ratios of 1:2, 2:3, or 3:4 were mixed to determine whether the ensemble periodicity and the component periodicities could be heard (Warren & Bashford, 1981). It was found that, while the ensemble periodicity (or waveform repetition rate) with the relative frequency of unity was dominant for each of the three ratios used, it also was possible for listeners to hear each of the harmonically related repetition frequencies.

Multiple harmonic frequencies can be teased apart in the pitch range as well. The first eight harmonics of a complex tone can each be detected (Plomp, 1964; Plomp & Mimpen, 1968), and this ability generally is attributed to place mechanisms based on spatial resolution along the basilar membrane. However, the perceptual resolution of harmonically related complex patterns each stimulating the same cochlear loci indicates that temporal analysis can separate multiple repetition frequencies.

Are there other infrapitch analogs of pitch range phenomena? Recent experiments have indicated that a number of effects perceived in the pitch range continue to be heard at infratonal repetition frequencies. Some of these studies will be described, and their implications for theory discussed.

ECHO PITCH AND INFRAPITCH ECHO

When a noise is added to itself after a delay of τ sec, an "echo pitch" is heard with a pitch equal to $1/\tau$ Hz for values of τ from 2×10^{-2} through 5×10^{-4} sec (pitches from 50 through 2,000 Hz; see Bilsen & Ritsma, 1969/70). Echo pitch is known by several other names including time-difference tone, reflection tone, time-separation pitch, repetition pitch, and rippled-noise pitch. This last name refers to its rippled power spectrum with peaks occurring at integral multiples of $1/\tau$ Hz (see Fig. 3.14A). While the rippled power spectrum shown corresponds to a mixture of undelayed and delayed noise having equal amplitudes, a pitch can still be heard for differences in intensity up to about 20 dB between the delayed and undelayed sounds (Yost & Hill, 1978). Theories proposed to explain echo pitch generally involve analyses based on the spacing of spectral peaks at some stage of neural processing. The spectral information is conveyed by a sequence of stimulation maxima along the basilar membrane as with complex tones but, while tones produce a line spectrum, the single acoustic restatements of echo pitch produce the band spectrum shown in figure 3.14A. According to spectral theories, the pitch heard for noise mixed with its echo corresponds to the fundamental of the harmonic series of peaks at $1/\tau$ Hz.

There is evidence that temporal information may contribute to echo pitch. Bilsen and Ritsma (1969/70) reported that, when the stimulus shown in figure 3.14A was band-pass filtered so that "roughly one spectral mountain" remained, a pitch of $1/\tau$ Hz was heard for each of the single spectral mountains up to at least the fourth or fifth peak. Similar observations for the pitch of band-pass filtered rippled power spectra were reported by Yost and Hill (1978). Since the different spectral mountains each have a common pitch of $1/\tau$ Hz when heard alone, temporal information concerning τ must be available at each locus. Figure 3.14A indicates that both spectral information, S, and temporal information, T, contribute to the echo pitch, P, of broad-band stimuli and that both types of cues indicate the same pitch value of $1/\tau$ Hz.

Warren, Bashford, and Wrightson (1980) reasoned that if temporal information could lead to detection of echo for delays producing pitch, it might be possible to detect an infrapitch echo at long delays for which spectral cues to repetition are absent. When this idea was tested, it was found that subjects could detect delays as long as 0.5 second (infrapitch iterance of 2 Hz). This long echo delay has spectral peaks separated by only 2 Hz, a spacing much too close to permit resolution along the basilar membrane, so that infrapitch echo could only be detected by information provided through temporal analysis. Infrapitch echo resembled infrapitch RGNs as described by Guttman and Julesz (1963), but was considerably fainter. As shown in figure 3.15, subjects were able to match the periods of echo delays quite accurately to the repetition rates of periodic sounds for values of τ from 0.5 through 0.01 second, corresponding to repetition frequencies from 2 Hz through 100 Hz respectively. (Matches were made on the basis of pitch iterance at 50 Hz and above, and on the basis of infrapitch iterance from 2 Hz through 20 Hz.) At frequencies of 5 Hz and below, it was possible for subjects to dispense with a matching stimulus, and also indicate accurately the repetition period of infrapitch echo directly by tapping a response key.

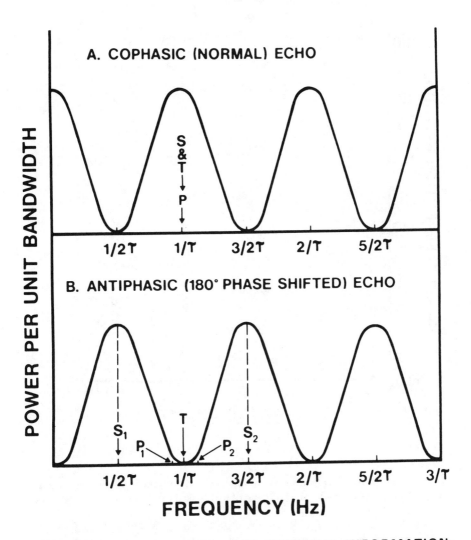

τ IS ECHO DELAY IN SEC; S IS SPECTRAL INFORMATION; T IS TEMPORAL INFORMATION; P IS ECHO PITCH

Fig. 3.14. Rippled power spectra produced by adding a delayed restatement of broad-band noise to itself. Spectral and temporal information agree in part A (based on normal or cophasic echo), but they conflict in part B (based on polarity inverted or antiphasic echo). The two pitches of antiphasic echo (P_1 and P_2) are considered to result from a conflict between temporal information (T) corresponding to a pitch of $1/\tau$ Hz, and spectral information (S_1 and S_2) from two flanking spectral peaks corresponding to pitches of $1/2\tau$ Hz and $3/2\tau$ Hz. See text for further information.

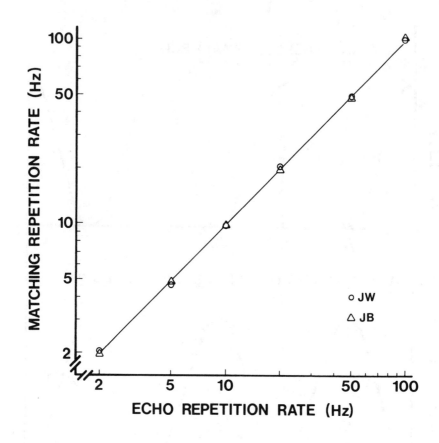

Fig. 3.15. Apparent repetition rate of noise mixed with its echo. Judgments of 50 and 100 Hz were made on the basis of pitch, and judgments of 2, 5, 10, and 20 Hz on the basis of infrapitch.

Source: R.M. Warren, J.A. Bashford, Jr., and J.M. Wrightson, "Infrapitch Echo," *Journal of the Acoustical Society of America* **68** (1980): 1301-05.

The nature of the infrapitch temporal analysis used for noise mixed with its echo may be clarified if we compare it with the infrapitch iterance of RGNs. We have seen that continued repetition of a segment of Gaussian noise A (that is, AAA...) can be detected readily for periods of A as long as 1 or 2 seconds (Guttman & Julesz, 1963). In preliminary experiments, Warren, Bashford, and Wrightson (1980) found that multiple repetitions of the same waveform were not required. If a 500 msec segment of noise (A) was repeated a single time, followed by a second 500 msec segment of noise (B) repeated once, then a third 500 msec segment of noise (C) repeated once, etc., to produce the stimulus AABBCC..., listeners could detect such a "pure" echo based on these single repetitions with somewhat greater ease than they could detect mixed infrapitch echo. The mixed infrapitch echo can be considered to have the composition A+B, B+C, C+D, D+E,..., where each letter corresponds to an independent noise segment. It can be seen that on the first appearance of C it is mixed with noise segment B, and on its single reappearance it is mixed with noise segment D. A mechanism is required for the extraction of temporal information corresponding to C from two uncorrelated maskers. A relatively simple mechanism involving recognition of the restatement of exceptional features associated with C might work for pure echo, but would not work for mixed echo. Different exceptional features would be created with the mixture of C with B, and of C with D, and any unique characteristics of C by itself would be changed, and changed differently by its mixture with B and its mixture with D. A mechanism used for detection of infrapitch mixed echo needs to be capable of recognizing masked single repetitions of long-period random patterns, a rather formidable task indicating considerable analytical power.

Reversing the polarity of the delayed noise (phase shifting by 180° to produce "antiphasic" echo) produced no noticeable difference at infrapitch delays. Repetition could be heard with equal ease for antiphasic and cophasic addition, and the apparent repetition frequency was $1/\tau$ Hz in both cases (Warren, Bashford, & Wrightson, 1980), so that the complex temporal pattern analysis was insensitive to polarity inversion. However, it is known that inverting the echo polarity in the pitch range produces a marked effect: antiphasic echo pitch is weaker and has two simultaneous pitches, one about 10 percent higher and one about 10 percent lower than cophasic echo with the same delay (Bilsen, 1970; Fourcin, 1965; Yost, Hill, & Perez-Falcon, 1978). Warren, Bashford, and Wrightson found that the change from polarity insensitivity to polarity sensitivity occurred at about $\tau = 0.025$ sec (40 Hz), which corresponds closely to the lower limit for neural place analysis (see chapter 1).

The pitch heard for antiphasic echo is troublesome for conventional pitch theories, since the double pitches of $1/0.9\tau$ and $1/1.1\tau$ Hz are centered on the spectral trough of $1/\tau$ Hz (see Fig. 3.14B). Bilsen and Goldstein (1974) and Bilsen (1977) attempted to account for this problem by considering that the auditory system constructs a "central spectrum" in which the fourth and fifth spectral peaks of an antiphasic echo spectrum are used by a central pitch extractor to calculate a fundamental corresponding to a successive harmonic (cophasic) echo spectrum. This calculation leads to two "pseudofundamentals" corresponding to the double antiphasic echo pitch perceived by listeners. It was considered that the central pitch extractor operating on the central spectrum produced by normal or cophasic echo uses only the third, fourth, and fifth peaks to calculate (in this case, accurately) the fundamental of the harmonic sequence of peaks corresponding to the pitch heard. However, this spectral model cannot handle the perception of infrapitch echo since the peaks of the acoustic power spectrum are too closely spaced to be resolved by the auditory system.

Warren, Bashford, and Wrightson (1980) suggested a different basis for the double pitch of antiphasic echo. They considered that ambiguity resulted from a conflict between temporal and spectral cues to pitch. While temporal cues indicate a repetition period equal to the echo delay of τ sec and corresponding to a pitch of $1/\tau$ Hz (shown in Fig. 3.14B as the temporal cue T), this frequency, as can be seen, corresponds to a spectral trough. A strictly spectral analysis should lead to a pitch of $1/2\tau$ Hz for antiphasic echo in keeping with the first peak in the rippled power spectrum (shown as spectral pitch S_1). Conflict of spectral and temporal analyses would then produce a compromise pitch indicated by P_1. The other neighboring spectral peak, S_2 (equal to $3/2\tau$ Hz), also would conflict with temporal analysis (and with the compromise pitch P_1), resulting in a second compromise pitch, P_2. These compromise pitches associated with the conflicting cues of antiphasic echo are weaker than cophasic echo pitch for which, as shown in figure 3.14A, the results of spectral analysis (S) and temporal analysis (T) coincide and reinforce each other at $1/\tau$ Hz. At infrapitch echo delays, spectral resolution of peaks is no longer possible. When both cophasic and antiphasic infrapitch echo have the same delay time of τ sec, the apparent frequency is based solely upon the delay time, and is $1/\tau$ Hz for each.

If, as suggested, a conflict between temporal and place cues to echo pitch is produced by the polarity inversion of antiphasic echo, then it may be possible to demonstrate an analogous conflict in pitch using strictly periodic stimuli. When a waveform is repeated with alternate statements inverted in polarity, a polarity insensitive temporal analysis should indicate a pitch twice that corresponding to the waveform repetition frequency (and the spectral fundamental). We shall see in the next section that conflicting pitches can be produced by periodic sounds with alternating polarity.

PERIODIC SIGNALS WITH ALTERNATING POLARITY

Warren and Wrightson (1981) used noise segments as model periodic waveforms, and determined the apparent frequency when alternate statements of the waveform were reversed in polarity. These stimuli had the form A_0, A_π, A_0, A_π,... in which A_0 represents a waveform derived from noise, and A_π the same waveform which has been inverted in polarity (that is, phase-shifted by 180° or π radians). The overall repetition frequencies employed in the study ranged from 2 Hz through 1,935 Hz. An illustration of a stimulus waveform is given in figure 3.16 for a 200 Hz signal.

If the duration of A_0 is $\tau/2$ sec, then the waveform repetition period corresponding to $(A_0 + A_\pi)$ is τ sec, and the fundamental frequency is $1/\tau$ Hz. As with all periodic sounds consisting of segments alternating in polarity but otherwise equivalent (square waves, symmetrical triangle waves, alternating polarity pulse trains, etc.), the spectrum contains only odd-numbered harmonics, so that the component frequencies are $1/\tau$, $3/\tau$, $5/\tau$, ... Hz.

The results, obtained when the apparent frequencies of iterated noise segments in the tonal and infratonal frequency ranges were matched using

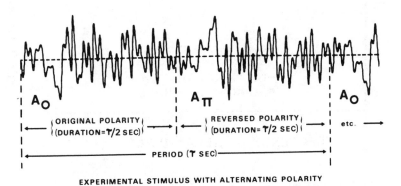

POLARITY REVERSAL OF NOISE SEGMENT

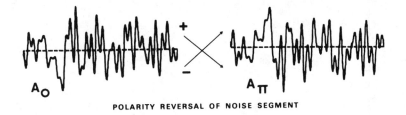

EXPERIMENTAL STIMULUS WITH ALTERNATING POLARITY

Fig. 3.16. Model randomly derived waveforms with alternating polarity. The overall period of τ sec consists of two segments each of $1/2\tau$ sec duration, each half-period representing a polarity inverted version of the other. This stimulus can produce conflicting temporal and spectral cues to iterance.
Source: R.M. Warren and J.M. Wrightson, "Stimuli Producing Conflicting Temporal and Spectral Cues to Frequency," *Journal of the Acoustical Society of America* 70 (1981): 1020-24.

adjustable unipolar pulse trains, are shown in figure 3.17. Values obtained for the iterated alternating polarity waveforms are indicated by squares, and values obtained for noise segments repeated without polarity inversions (used as an experimental control to determine accuracy of frequency matching) are indicated by circles.

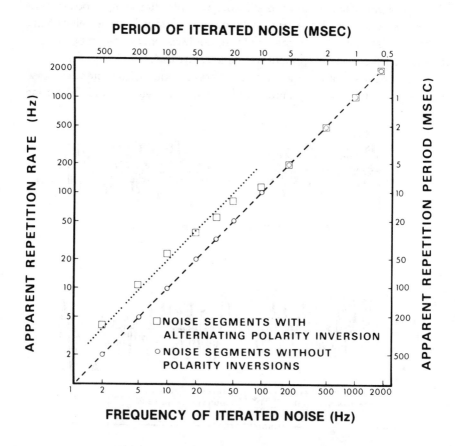

Fig. 3.17. Apparent repetition rates of iterated noise segments with and without polarity inversion of alternate statements. The diagonal dashed line represents apparent frequencies equal to the waveform repetition frequencies (and the spectral fundamentals). The dotted diagonal line represents polarity-insensitive apparent frequencies one octave higher than the waveform repetition frequencies.

Source: R.M. Warren and J.M. Wrightson, "Stimuli Producing Conflicting Temporal and Spectral Cues to Frequency," *Journal of the Acoustical Society of America* 70 (1981): 1020-24.

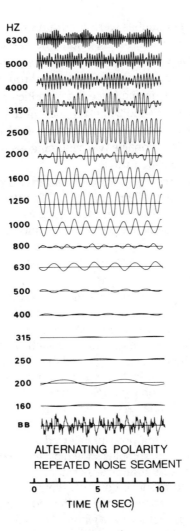

Fig. 3.18. Illustration of the nature of basilar membrane responses to a model periodic waveform with alternating polarity. The 200 Hz alternating polarity noise segment, shown in the bottom of the figure in broad-band form (as BB), has an overall period of 5 msec with successive 2.5 msec segments identical except for polarity inversion. As in figures 3.9 and 3.11 based on the same set of 1/3-octave filters (center frequencies shown on the left), response curves show spectral resolution at the lower center frequencies, and complex periodic waveforms at the higher. Examination of the responses of filters with center frequencies of 2,000 Hz and above indicates that their responses to successive 2.5 msec segments are generally similar in structure, suggesting a waveform repetition frequency of 400 Hz.

It can be seen that matches were accurate for the control stimuli at all frequencies. However, the alternating polarity noise segments were matched with unipolar pulse trains of the same repetition frequency only at 200 Hz and above. At infratonal frequencies from 2 Hz through 20 Hz, they were matched with pulse trains having twice the repetition frequency. Within the low pitch range between 20 and 200 Hz, apparent frequency represented a compromise between the polarity-insensitive infrapitch mode and the spectral high-pitch mode. Occasionally, two simultaneous pitches were reported for a stimulus in this transition range.

Figure 3.18 illustrates the nature of patterns produced by a 200 Hz alternating polarity stimulus when a series of 1/3-octave filters were used to simulate critical bands on the basilar membrane as in figures 3.9 and 3.11. It can be seen that the fundamental and lower harmonics are resolved by this model of basilar membrane filtering. At center frequencies of the filter above about 1,000 Hz, harmonic components interact to generate iterated complex patterns.

While both complex patterns and spectral resolution can be seen for the 200 Hz stimulus in figure 3.18, both cues to acoustic repetition would not be available throughout the range of repetition frequencies used by Warren and Wrightson. When listeners received the infrapitch alternating polarity noise segment having a frequency of 2 Hz (period of 0.5 sec), the close spacing of successive harmonics ensured that many harmonics were present within each critical band, so that only complex temporal patterns were produced along the basilar membrane. As shown in figure 3.17, listeners heard a repetition frequency of $2/\tau$ or 4 Hz with this 2 Hz stimulus, indicating perceptual equivalence of the polarity inverted waveforms. In contrast, the 1,935 Hz alternating polarity stimulus should permit spectral resolution of the fundamental and most of the audible harmonics, without any appreciable harmonic interaction to produce complex temporal patterns. As shown in figure 3.17, the 1,935 Hz stimulus had a pitch corresponding to $1/\tau$ Hz (its fundamental frequency). Somewhere within the pitch range, a transition between the two analytical modes should occur, with evidence of analyses corresponding to both $2/\tau$ Hz and $1/\tau$ Hz. Figure 3.17 shows that this ambiguity was found for frequencies greater than 20 Hz and less than 200 Hz.

The simulation of basilar membrane excitation shown in figure 3.18 indicates that the 200 Hz alternating polarity signal has information concerning individual harmonic components available for both place analysis and simple phase-locked period analysis at lower critical bands and, in addition, polarity insensitive complex pattern information at higher critical bands. It appears that the information concerning the fundamental frequency may suppress (or dominate) the polarity insensitive temporal information. If this reasoning is correct, then high-pass filtering of the 200 Hz stimulus should remove the perceptually dominant information concerning the low spectral harmonics, and so cause a doubling in apparent frequency. This was found to be the case. When the 200 Hz stimulus shown in figure 3.18 was high-pass filtered at 2,000 Hz by Warren and Wrightson, the apparent frequency changed from 200 Hz to 400 Hz.

An examination of figure 3.18 suggests a possible basis for the perceptual insensitivity to polarity inversion for complex pattern cues. The broad-band tracing at the bottom of the figure shows a clear change (a polarity inversion) of the waveform pattern every 2.5 msec. However, changes corresponding to the phase-shift of π radians are much less clear for the filtered complex waveform patterns generated through interaction of neighboring harmonics within 1/3-octave bands. Close inspection of such patterns at the higher band-pass filter settings shows that successive 2.5 msec segments have details of fine structure (in terms of both amplitude of peaks and time intervals between successive peaks) which are changed by polarity inversion, but these differences are quite small. While the filtering occurring within the ear prior to stimulation of auditory nerve fibers (see chapter 1) is, of course, not identical to the simulation depicted in figure 3.18, the simulation does suggest that perceptual equivalence of polarity inverted complex patterns may be attributable to the effects of acoustic filtering.

If the segregation of closely spaced neighboring harmonics by spectral filtering minimizes the effect of a π radian (180°) phase shift, we would expect a similar effect when complex waveforms are shifted through other phase angles. This was found to be the case. While oscilloscope tracings showed that the broad-band waveform changed considerably when a 2.5 msec noise segment was repeated with alternate statements shifted through any phase angle greater than a few degrees, the successive 2.5 msec complex patterns for the 1/3-octave bands containing several higher harmonics appeared to be quite similar. When listeners heard a noise segment repeated at infratonal frequencies with alternate statements shifted by any particular phase angle, the apparent repetition frequency was insensitive to the changes in phase. Thus, when a 250 msec segment of noise was repeated with alternate statements shifted by 180°, 90°, 57°, or any other phase angle, the repetition frequency heard was always 4 Hz. Also, when listeners were allowed to switch at will between a 4 Hz iterated noise segment and a phase-shifted version of the same stimulus, the two repeated waveforms were indistinguishable at all phase angles. (A pair of independently generated iterated noise segments were readily distinguished under these conditions.) These observations suggest that the polarity insensitivity of complex pattern perception may be a special case of the insensitivity of this type of temporal analysis to shifting of acoustic waveforms by any phase angle.

Perception of alternating polarity noise segments is of interest for two reasons: (1) this stimulus can produce a highly unusual conflict between modes of frequency analysis—usually when more than one mechanism for perceiving iterance is present, they are in agreement, and it is not possible to establish the relative importance of each; and (2) since repeated noise segments are considered as model stimuli, the results obtained should be applicable to other waveforms repeated with alternating polarity and, in particular, can help explain observations which have been reported for alternating polarity pulse trains.

Alternating Polarity Pulse Trains

Flanagan and Guttman (1960a) were the first to note that the apparent pitch of alternating polarity pulse trains with frequencies of 32 Hz (64 pulses per sec) or less were determined by the pulse rate, while the apparent pitch of alternating polarity pulse trains with frequencies of 210 Hz (420 pulses per sec) or more corresponded to the spectral fundamental (see Fig. 3.19). Between these frequencies, the pitch of the alternating polarity pulse trains was ambiguous, with the combined judgments of their subjects intermediate between values corresponding to spectral matching and to pulse-rate matching. They attributed the pulse-rate matching mode to the ability of the basilar membrane to resolve the separate pulses in time, stating that this mode required that each place along the basilar membrane receive temporally discrete pulses (Flanagan & Guttman, 1960a, 1960b; Guttman & Flanagan, 1964). It was considered that when pulses became temporally blurred with one pulse beginning before movement produced by the preceding pulse ended, then pulse-rate matching was lost. High-pass filtering at a few kiloHertz raised the upper limit of the pitch-matching mode, and this was attributed to removal of components which did not produce temporally resolved pulses on the basilar membrane (Flanagan, 1972, pp. 128-130; Guttman & Flanagan, 1964). However, explanations in terms of special pulsate characteristics do not explain why similar rules are followed by nonpulsate stimuli (see Fig. 3.17). It seems, rather, that the observations concerning apparent frequency of alternating polarity pulse trains represent the application of a general rule to a specific waveform.

PITCHES PRODUCED BY DICHOTIC INTERACTIONS

Houtsma and Goldstein (1972) presented two adjacent harmonics of a missing fundamental simultaneously for a duration of 500 msec, followed 250 msec later by a second 500 msec stimulus also consisting of two adjacent harmonics but with a different missing fundamental. These two missing fundamentals

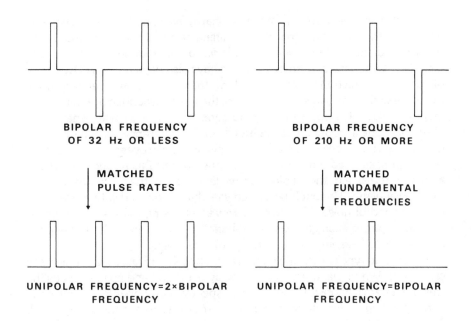

Fig. 3.19. Alternating polarity pulse trains and unipolar pulse trains judged to be matched in pitch. At fundamental spectral frequencies of 32 Hz or less, pulse trains with alternating polarity were matched with unipolar pulse trains on the basis of pulse rate (pulses per second). At fundamental spectral frequencies of 210 Hz or more, the alternating polarity pulse trains were matched with unipolar pulse trains on the basis of the spectral fundamental. At intermediate repetition frequencies, both modes of pitch matching occurred, resulting in two pitches for alternating polarity pulse trains.
Source: R.M. Warren and J.M. Wrightson, "Stimuli Producing Conflicting Temporal and Spectral Cues to Frequency," *Journal of the Acoustical Society of America* 70 (1981): 1020-24; based on data from J.L. Flanagan and N. Guttman, "On the Pitch of Periodic Pulses," *Journal of the Acoustical Society of America* 32 (1960): 1308-19.

together corresponded to one of eight possible musical intervals, and their musically trained subjects were required to identify the interval, or, as it was considered, the two-note "melody." Houtsma and Goldstein found that this task could be accomplished not only when each component of the two-harmonic stimulus producing a missing fundamental note was delivered simultaneously to the same ear (monaural stimulation) but also could be identified when one harmonic of the two-harmonic complex was delivered to one ear at the same time that the remaining harmonic was delivered to the other ear (dichotic stimulation). In addition to the creation of pitch through dichotic interactions of harmonics, there have also been reports of two types of rather faint dichotic pitches resulting from time delays between noise signals reaching the two ears. The first of these was described by Cramer and Huggins (1958). They presented broad-band noise from a single generator to both ears, but introduced an interaural phase difference for a narrow frequency band lying below 1,000 Hz. This phase change over a small frequency range approximated a fixed time delay and caused this frequency band to appear at the side of the leading ear, while the rest of the noise was heard at the medial plane. The pitch perceived was that associated with the laterally isolated band of noise. However, there was no monaural spectral information: the input to each ear was broad-band noise with no pitch, so that pitch emerged only following binaural temporal processing.

A second type of dichotic temporal pitch has been discussed earlier (see chapter 2). When the interaural time delay of broad-band noise exceeds the limit for lateralization for some of the spectral components, a faint pitch corresponding in Hertz to the reciprocal of the delay in seconds can be heard. The limits of the range of interaural time delays reported to produce such pitch extend from about 3 msec through 50 msec, corresponding to about 300 through about 20 Hz (Bilsen & Goldstein, 1974; Fourcin, 1970; Warren, Bashford, & Wrightson, 1981).

The existence of these three types of dichotic pitches demonstrates that it is possible to generate pitch through binaural interactions when information received at each ear alone is insufficient to establish the pitch heard.

EAR DOMINANCE FOR PERCEPTION OF PITCH

While Houtsma and Goldstein (1972) demonstrated that dichotic information involving different pitches can be integrated to produce a third pitch, there have been experiments demonstrating that under some conditions there is a perceptual suppression of one of two tones presented dichotically. Deutsch has reported a number of illusions in which a lateral dominance is observed for the perception of different tones delivered to each ear simultaneously (Deutsch, 1974, 1975; Deutsch & Roll, 1976). She has observed that the dominant pitch is sometimes mislateralized, and has concluded that information concerning pitch and lateralization can be disassociated and processed independently at some stage (Deutsch,1981). Efron and Yund (1976) have reported that lateral dominance for "dichotic chords" is not like that for monaural chords: for the monaural condition, relative intensities strongly influence the contribution of each component to perception; for the dichotic condition, there is a wide range of intensity mismatch over which lateral advantage can be maintained for a fainter tone.

MUSICAL PITCH AND
MUSICAL INFRAPITCH (RHYTHM)

Musical pitch spans about seven octaves. The lowest note of a bass viol at 41 Hz represents the lower limit, and the highest note of a piccolo at about 4,500 Hz represents the upper limit of orchestral instruments. Of course, harmonics of the fundamental frequencies corresponding to musical notes may be present up to the 16,000 or 20,000 Hz limit of hearing, and enter into determining the quality of a tone. But why the rather low upper frequency limit for musical pitch? One possibility is that qualities of musical sounds depend to a large extent on their harmonic structure, and since there is little headroom left for audible harmonics above 4,500 Hz, these high pitches are not used in music and so seem amelodic. Another possibility is that place and simple pattern periodicity information occur together only from about 50 through 5,000 Hz (see Fig. 3.12), and melodic appreciation requires both types of information.

Musical intervals correspond to fixed ratios between the frequencies of notes. The basic unit is the octave (2:1) which is used in virtually all cultures having well-developed musical systems (see Helmholtz, 1877). The division of the octave into smaller intervals is culture-dependent. The music used in Western culture employs intervals for which the fundamental frequencies stand in the ratio of small integers: for example, fifths (frequency ratio of 3:2), minor thirds (frequency ratio of 6:5), major thirds (frequency ratio of 5:4). A pair of notes corresponding to one of these intervals seems consonant when sounded simultaneously by musical instruments, and one reason for this harmonious or consonant relation could involve the matching of frequencies for some of the harmonics from each note. Interestingly, the rules for consonance of complex tones do not seem to apply for pure tones. In a study by Plomp and Levelt (1965), pure tones were generally rated as dissonant when they fell within the same critical band, and consonant when they were separated by more than a critical band. The sinusoidal tones falling within a single critical band produce beats and "roughness" which appear to be associated with dissonance, while the consonant sinusoidal tones stimulating nonoverlapping loci are each smooth-sounding.

The ability to recognize musical notes or intervals is limited to notes below the upper limit of orchestral instruments. Bachem (1948) used subjects with absolute pitch (the ability to identify a note heard alone without the help of a reference note), and found that they could not identify notes above the orchestral limit. He stated that these subjects reported that the concept of musical pitch seemed to be without meaning at these high frequencies. In another experiment, Ward (1954) used musicians, each of whom played at least two instruments, and had them estimate the octaves of pure tones. While this task was done with accuracy within the musical range by all, when the frequency was raised above the highest note of a piccolo, only two of the nine subjects could estimate octaves. Ward found out that these two had experience with oscillators generating pure tones, and determined that they could estimate octaves accurately up to the limit of audibility of sinusoidal tones. Hence, it appears that training may extend the upper limit of musical interval recognition.

Rhythm in music involves the repetition of auditory patterns at infratonal frequencies. It appears that music plays with acoustic repetition (and systematic variations from strict repetition) not only in the pitch range, but in the infrapitch range as well. Music can involve multiple infratonal periodicities having considerable complexity: African polyrhythms use long-period sequences of percussive sounds which can contain several harmonically related rhythmic frequencies, and listeners can attend either to the ensemble periodicity or to one or another of the rhythmic components. However, unlike the case with mixed infratonal RGNs, the individual rhythmic percussive lines can be followed even when they deviate from harmonic relations with other lines: some African music uses "additive polyrhythms" in which component inharmonic periodicities are each perceived (see Sachs, 1953), while work by Warren and Bashford (1981) has shown that mixing of inharmonic infratonal RGNs inhibits the detection of any periodicity.

Complex Beats: Integration of Different Infrapitch Periodicities at Different Cochlear Loci

Both polyrhythms and superimposed harmonically related RGNs demonstrate that differentiation of multiple infratonal periodicities can take place when these periodicities stimulate a common broad location on the basilar membrane. Recent experiments have shown that, in addition to this ability to analyze or tease apart simultaneous periodicities, we also possess the converse ability to synthesize or integrate infratonal periodicities even when they stimulate separate loci on the basilar membrane. Thus, it has been reported that when two uncorrelated tonal RGNs—one at 199 Hz and one at 201 Hz—were superimposed and low-pass filtered at 8,100 Hz, a single beat rate of 2 Hz was heard, despite the fact that each of the 40 harmonics of one RGN interacted with the corresponding harmonic of the other to produce a harmonic sequence of beat rates (a "complex beat") with 40 components (2, 4, 6, 8, ... 80 Hz) (Warren, 1978). After filtering off the fundamental tonal frequencies (and removing the 2 Hz beat rate), an ensemble 2 Hz periodicity was still heard. Further experiments used three to five pairs of beating sinusoidal tones to generate complex beats. By adjusting the frequency difference between members of a tone pair, any desired beat rate could be produced; and, by adjusting the center frequency of each tone pair, the individual beat rates could be delivered to any frequency-sensitive place on the basilar membrane.

This manipulation of individual beat rates, each stimulating a different place on the basilar membrane, permitted examination of the ability of listeners to combine temporal information originating at different loci and carried by separate groups of auditory nerve fibers. It was observed that integration of the infratonal temporal information took place under all conditions employed, including those involving nonoverlapping, widely separated positions on the basilar membrane. Even when the fundamental rate of the complex beat was missing, the ensemble or pooled infratonal periodicity corresponding to the missing fundamental beat rate was heard.

Effects of Deviations from Strict Infrapitch Periodicity

While the ability to recognize repetition (and deviation from exact repetition) of auditory patterns is used for perception of rhythm and identification of melodic themes, this ability enters into other aspects of musical perception in a less obvious fashion. Sustained notes produced by a musical instrument or a singer are not steady, but fluctuate appreciably in intensity and frequency. While quasi-periodic variations at infratonal frequencies such as vibrato or tremelo are quite deliberate and noticeable, there are other fluctuations not detectable as such, but rather as a "natural" quality. When single periods are excised from a recording of any musical instrument playing a particular note and iterated to produce a note unchanging in intensity and pitch, the instrument is no longer identifiable (unless it happens to be an organ). Robert Moog has stated on several occasions that all instruments sound like an organ when a single period is excised and repeated without change. He believes that, "It is an inescapable fact that instruments sound the way they do because of the ways the waveform changes." (Dr. Moog, personal communication.)

The ability to detect slight fluctuations in amplitude and frequency can be demonstrated when a one second segment of a "steady" note produced by a musical instrument or a voice is recycled on a digital delay line. It appears that listeners can perceive that loudness and pitch are fluctuating regularly when the variations are made periodic; when aperiodic, these fluctuations become part of the characteristic quality of the sound.

SOME RECENT MODELS FOR THE PITCH OF COMPLEX TONES

A number of theories have considered that spatial patterning of stimulated regions along the basilar membrane determines the pitch heard. Thurlow (1963) has suggested that there can be vocal mediation of the spatial patterning in which the listener either covertly or overtly matches the pitch of the sound with his or her own production of a periodic vocal sound having matching harmonic components. (This vocal mediation mechanism would be limited to the pitch range of voice.) Whitfield (1970) considered that peripheral spatial resolution leads to corresponding patterns of activity of discrete groups of neural units at more central locations, and that these patterns are responsible for pitch. Whitfield stated that experience with complex harmonic patterns could serve as the basis for pitch judgments; and that, even when components such as the fundamental are missing, the remaining information would be sufficient for recognition of the overall pattern and identification of the fundamental pitch.

Terhardt (1974) proposed a learning-matrix model for extracting "virtual pitch" through a comparison of a complex tone with traces acquired through experience with other complex tones. He considered that, over one's lifetime, individual harmonic components are each associated with subharmonics, and, when the matrix of subharmonics corresponding to a group of component frequencies interact, they produce a "virtual" low pitch characteristic of the complex.

Wightman's (1973) pattern-transformation model considers that the first stage in pitch processing is a rough spectral analysis accomplished through the peripheral auditory system, followed by a Fourier transform of the spectrum, with the final stage corresponding to a pitch extractor which calculates the lowest maximum in the derived function.

Goldstein's (1973) optimum-processor model considers that resolved harmonics produce an approximate or "noisy" central representation of their frequencies. A central processor then computes the harmonic numbers of these components and derives from this the fundamental frequency which corresponds to the perceived pitch. Goldstein (1978) stated that, while cochlear filtering is an essential stage in auditory frequency analysis, neural time-following determines the precision of pitch judgments.

Each of these models was designed to deal only with pitch perception, and cannot be extended readily to handle perception of infrapitch iterance.

It would appear desirable to have a broader model or theory which can handle perception of acoustic iterance not only in a pitch range, but in the infrapitch range as well. Such a theory need not consider a single mechanism operating over the entire range of detectable iterance—indeed, as discussed earlier in this chapter, it appears probable that there are at least three mechanisms with overlapping frequency ranges used for detection of iterance.

4

The Measurement of Loudness and Pitch

SENSORY INPUT AND PERCEPTION

This chapter deals with some consequences of the twin principles that: (1) we are not aware of the nature of neurophysiological events and changes as such; and (2) sensation and perception are fundamentally equivalent, both involving the calibration of afferent input in terms of environmental correlates. The *sone* scale of loudness and the *mel* scale of pitch will be discussed, and evidence will be presented suggesting that these measures of sensation magnitude are disguised estimates of physical correlates.

While it seems reasonable to consider that the nature of sensory stimulation is primary, and that evaluation of external conditions and events based upon sensory input is an inference, in everyday life it often seems to be the other way around. That is, perception of objects and events appears to occur directly, while the nature of sensory stimulation leading to perception is inferred. In the previous discussion of auditory localization, we have seen how differences in acoustic input to the two ears are perceived in terms of associated external conditions and events without awareness of the aspects of sensory stimulation leading to this perception. Thus, when the sound radiated by a source reaches one ear before the other, listeners hear only a single sound located on the side of the leading ear: the lateral difference in time of stimulation can be inferred by those having some knowledge of acoustics, but even they perceive only one off-center sound. Also, we have seen that interaural spectral differences approximating those produced by the head and pinna for sources at different azimuths are perceived in an obligatory manner in terms of location rather than spectral mismatch.

Interpretation of sensory input in terms of environmental correlates is not, of course, unique to hearing. The disparity of the retinal images produced by perspective differences at the positions of the two eyes is not seen as a double image but, rather, in terms of the apparent distances of objects represented by these images. Perception of depth is accomplished effortlessly without any awareness of differences in the retinal images. It is an intellectual exercise of some difficulty to use the laws of perspective to reason that objects are closer than the fixation distance determined by ocular vergence if they produce a crossed binocular disparity (i.e., a shift to the left for the right eye and a shift to the right for the left eye), and that they are further than the fixation distance if they produce an opposite uncrossed disparity.

There is a related perceptual principle that aspects of sensory input which do not correspond to external events are difficult (and sometimes impossible) to detect. This principle appears to have received greater emphasis in studies dealing with vision than with hearing. Thus, the large visual gap or blind spot corresponding to the optic disc is quite difficult to perceive. Similarly, the shadows cast by retinal blood vessels can be seen by only some viewers, even after special training and use of optimal viewing conditions. In hearing, we know that contraction of intra-aural muscles (the stapedius and the tensor tympani) produces a considerable change in auditory stimulation (see chapter 1). Yet this alteration in sensory response is not perceived: the level of sensation appears fixed in accordance with the unchanging stimulus level, not the changing level of neural input.

In keeping with these observations, we shall see that when subjects are required to estimate relative loudness they cannot base their answers upon the quantitative nature of sensory processes. Instead, responses are based upon quantifiable physical dimensions familiar to subjects and associated with changes in stimulation.

THE HISTORY OF LOUDNESS MEASUREMENT

The measurement of sensory intensity has had a long history of controversy. Fechner (1860) was the first to attempt to relate sensory magnitude to physical intensity. His idea was simple: all just noticeable difference (jnd) steps are subjectively equal, and the magnitude of a particular sensation can be measured by adding up the number of jnd steps from threshold to the level of that sensation. Thus, a sensation 25 jnd steps above threshold would be half that corresponding to a sensation 50 jnd steps above threshold. Fechner claimed that if Weber's law was valid (this law states that the size of a jnd is equal to a constant times the stimulus intensity), then it was possible to integrate the number of jnd steps above threshold and obtain the logarithmic relation:

$$S = k \log I + C \qquad\qquad\qquad \text{(Eq. 4.1)}$$

where S is sensory magnitude, I is stimulus intensity, and both k and C are constants.

Fechner believed that sensory magnitude could be measured only indirectly through the summing of jnd steps. However, Plateau (1872) attempted to measure visual sensation directly by asking viewers to estimate relative magnitudes, and found that the same fraction of the standard level was judged half subjective magnitude at all levels of the standard stimulus. Plateau used this empirical rule that *equal stimulus ratios produce equal subjective ratios* to derive a power function, and suggested that for all sensory modalities:

$$S = kI^n \qquad\qquad\qquad\qquad\qquad (Eq.4.2)$$

where, as above, S equals sensory magnitude, I equals stimulus intensity, and both k and n are constants.

There were only a few early attempts to measure loudness, probably because of the difficulty in achieving accurate control of relative stimulus intensities. One method used involved the impulsive sound produced by a weight striking a metal plate, with intensity controlled by varying the distance the weight fell. Aside from the primitive nature of such a procedure compared with the refined methods then available for controlling visual intensity, there was another difficulty. This manner of controlling sound intensity created a clear image of the procedure associated with changing loudness, and it was found that subjects were influenced in their judgments of relative loudness by mental estimates of relative distances the weight dropped.

The first study of loudness using steady-state stimuli with accurate intensity control was carried out by Richardson and Ross (1930). Their stimuli were tones which were delivered through earphones. It was reported that loudness was a power function of the stimulus over the entire 80 dB range they employed. Different exponents were obtained for the power functions of the individual subjects, with a combined exponent of 0.25 for their group of 11 subjects. Following this pioneering work, a number of other loudness experiments were reported. The results obtained generally were complex empirical functions, with no attempt by the experimenters to suggest that there was a simple relationship between sensation intensity and stimulus intensity.

The results of these many studies were tabulated by S.S. Stevens in 1955. There was considerable variability in reports from individual laboratories for half-loudness judgments, with the attenuation required ranging from 2.1 dB (62 percent of the standard intensity) to 24 dB (0.4 percent of the standard intensity). The distribution of values reported was skewed, probably reflecting the intrinsic asymmetry of the response range, which was limited to zero dB attenuation of the standard at the upper end and threshold intensity (which could be as much as 80 or 90 dB below the standard level) at the lower end. Stevens, faced with this mass of discrepant data, took a bold simplifying step. He was nonevaluative, accepted all studies, and calculated the median value reported for half-loudness. This value (–10 dB) was assumed to hold at all standard levels and was used for constructing the *sone* scale of loudness. This *sone* scale was a power function having an exponent of 0.3. The last recommendation by Stevens (1972) was a change from –10 dB to –9 dB for half-loudness corresponding to the function:

$$L = kI^{0.33} \qquad \text{(Eq. 4.3)}$$

Stevens (1961) stated that sensory organs can be considered as transducers converting energy in the environment to neural form, and that the input-output relations of these tranducers determine the exponent of psychophysical functions. He maintained this position over the years, and in a book published shortly after his death (Stevens, 1975), he restated his belief that the nature of built-in neural responses was responsible for sensory power functions.

Little neurophysiological work in hearing has been reported relating the neurophysiological responses of receptors to the psychophysical power function. However, a number of attempts have been made to relate neurophysiological responses in vision to the psychophysical brightness function, with considerable disagreement among investigators working in neurophysiology concerning the success of such attempts. This controversy is beyond the scope of this chapter, but interested readers are referred to Hood and Finkelstein (1981), Mansfield (1981), Warren (1981a), and Wasserman (1981).

There also have been attempts to account for psychophysical power scales in terms of nonlinear use of numbers, and in terms of interactive and conjoint measures involving several variables. In addition, there have been those who deny that sensation can be measured: Tumarkin (1972) described the domain of psychophysics as a land of mystery and magic where bewitched psychophysicists seek to capture will-o'-the-wisps. These topics have been discussed fairly exhaustively in published commentaries accompanying a target article on measurement of sensation (Warren, 1981a). This article reviewed evidence from several sensory modalities (including hearing), and concluded that judgments of the magnitude of sensation appear to be based upon experience with correlated physical scales. Some of the evidence described for loudness will be discussed in the following sections.

APPARENT LOUDNESS AND ITS RELATION TO AUDITORY LOCALIZATION: THE PHYSICAL CORRELATE THEORY

We have seen in chapter 2 that intensity of sound is a major cue used by listeners to estimate the distance of a sound source. Early in this century, Gamble (1909) noted that changes in loudness and changes in distance seemed to be equivalent concepts for listeners hearing sounds at different intensities. She stated that "...judgments of 'nearer' and 'louder' and of 'farther' and 'softer' were practically interchangeable." Warren, Sersen, and Pores (1958) have suggested that familiarity with the manner in which sound stimuli change with distance provides the basis for judgments of "subjective" magnitude, so that half-loudness judgments are equivalent to estimates of the effect of doubling distance from the source. This suggestion was part of a general theory (the "physical correlate theory") which considers judgments of sensory magnitudes to be disguised estimates of physical magnitudes (Warren, 1958).

The specific consequences of the physical correlate (PC) theory for loudness judgments that have been put to experimental tests are the following:

1. Estimates of half-loudness and estimates of the effect of doubling the distance from the source should be equivalent when made under the same listening conditions by separate groups of subjects.
2. Under conditions designed to facilitate accurate estimates of the change in intensity with distance, both twice-distance and half-loudness judgments should be predictable from the inverse square law governing intensity changes with distance.
3. Since the degree of reverberation as well as intensity can change the apparent distance of a sound (see chapter 2), it should be possible to modify apparent loudness in a predictable fashion by manipulation of reverberation.
4. People can operate not only as sound receivers but as generators of sound as well. Subjects should be capable of adjusting the level of self-generated sounds to compensate for changes in intensity reaching a target as its distance is varied. Reduction of self-generated sound to half-loudness should correspond to the change required for maintenance of a fixed level at a target when its distance is halved.
5. It should be possible to create new loudness functions by providing listeners with experience correlating new physical scales with changes in level of stimulation. Specifically, familiarity with measurement of intensity using sound-level meters should lead to a loudness scale isomorphic with the deciBel scale.

As we shall see, each of these anticipated consequences of the physical correlate theory has experimental support.

Equivalence of Half-Loudness and Twice-Distance Estimates

Warren, Sersen, and Pores (1958) found that subjects asked to estimate half-loudness chose the same attenuation selected by a second group of subjects asked to estimate the effect of doubling distance from the source. Stevens and Guirao (1962) confirmed these findings: their subjects also selected the same attenuation for twice-distance and for half-loudness (twice softness) estimates.

Agreement of Half-Loudness with the Inverse Square Law

As a reasonably close approximation, sounds reaching a listener directly from a source follow the inverse square law (see chapter 2), so that, under conditions minimizing errors in estimating the effect of distance upon intensity, one-quarter intensity or –6 dB should (according to PC theory) correspond to both twice-apparent distance and half-loudness. However, Stevens' (1972) last recommendation based on a number of studies was that –9 dB corresponds to half-loudness. It has been suggested by Warren (1970a) that systematic biases toward overestimating attenuation were present in most loudness experiments, but that it might be possible to design bias-free conditions.

We have seen that when Stevens (1955) proposed his *sone* power function for loudness, he pooled widely discrepant experimental values for half-loudness from different laboratories which ranged from –2.1 dB to –24 dB. This variability reflects a great sensitivity to experimentally induced biases. The range of comparisons is known to influence judgments, and a strong bias toward selecting values for half-loudness in the middle of the available range has been reported by Garner (1954). Also, an immediately prior judgment has a large "transfer" effect upon apparent loudness, and attempts to compensate for this by a balanced experimental design may not succeed because of asymmetrical transfer effects (Poulton & Freeman, 1966). In addition to these general biasing effects, there are a number of other conditions associated with particular psychophysical methods capable of exerting strong influence upon loudness judgments. (See Warren, 1977a, for discussion.)

The "bias-free" conditions designed to test PC theory critically involved single-loudness judgments of untrained subjects unfamiliar with psychophysical theory and experiments. Subjects were presented with only two sound intensities: the standard or reference level, and the comparison level used for judging relative loudness. Subjects could switch between the two levels at will. After making their single loudness judgment, they were dismissed and not used as subjects again. Steady sounds (tones and white noise) were used to minimize the possible influence of reverberation cues to relative distance. (The effect of reverberation on loudness is discussed in the following section.) A separate group of 30 subjects was used with each pair of stimuli, so that this procedure had the practical disadvantage of requiring large numbers of subjects (over 3,000 listeners were employed in these loudness experiments). Since there is a bias toward selecting values in the middle of the response range, this single judgment procedure can provide bias-free judgments only for the comparison level corresponding to the middle of the response range of a monotonic loudness function.

Numerical loudness judgments were obtained for various attenuations of a 1,000 Hz tone relative to an 85 dB standard level assigned a loudness of 100 (Warren, 1970a). Results are shown in figure 4.1. Each data point corresponds to the mean of judgments by 30 subjects, and the filled data points represent values that are not significantly different from the loudness of 50 (which is free from response-range bias). It can be seen that the intersection of the monotonic loudness function with the midrange value of 50 occurred at a 6 dB attenuation, in keeping with PC theory. Other experiments (not shown in Fig. 4.1) demonstrated that a 6 dB attenuation corresponded to half-loudness of a 1,000 Hz tone for the range of moderate standard levels from 45 through 92 dB,and that this attenuation also corresponded to half-loudness for tones at other frequencies (250 through 6,000 Hz) presented at moderate intensities (Warren, 1970a). Another series of experiments used Gaussian noise rather than tones (Warren, 1973a). Figure 4.1 shows that –6 dB corresponded to half-loudness of an 85 dB Gaussian noise for presentation both through headphones and over loudspeakers. Loudspeakers were not used with tones because of standing waves associated with the reflection of steady-state tones from surfaces, even in sound-treated audiometric rooms. These standing waves result in differences in intensity at the two ears and changes in monaural intensity with relatively slight head movements. Standing waves are not established for the constantly changing waveform of noise, and it can be seen in figure 4.1 that with both headphones and loudspeakers the attenuation of –6 dB corresponding to theory was found for the midrange value of 50. Other experiments (not shown in the figure) demonstrated that, as in the case of tones, –6 dB corresponded to half-loudness of noise over the middle or moderate range of standard levels from 45 through 95 dB (Warren, 1973a).

In another experiment measuring the loudness of noise, subjects listening through headphones were given a line labeled "louder sound" at one end and "silence" at the other, and they indicated the loudness of a fainter comparison sound relative to an 85 dB standard by the position of a mark made upon this line (Warren, 1973a). Responses were scored as percentage of the distance from the "silent" end to the "louder sound" end. The results

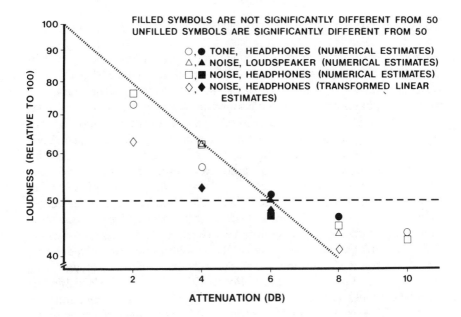

Fig. 4.1. Loudness judgments for different attenuations of a 1,000 Hz tone and of Gaussian noise relative to 85 dB SPL standards. Numerical judgments, relative to the assigned loudness value of 100 for the standards, are shown for both tone and noise. In addition, transformed linear estimates, based on marks on a line labeled "silence" at one end and "louder sound" at the other, are shown for noise (see text for further description). The diagonal dotted line corresponds to loudness proportional to the square root of the stimulus intensity, and the horizontal dashed line corresponds to the mid-range value of 50 free from asymmetrical response bias. The intersection of these lines (loudness of 50, 6 dB attenuation) represents conditions testing the physical correlate theory. Each data point corresponds to the mean of first judgments from a separate group of 30 subjects.

Source: Figure from R. M. Warren, "Measurement of Sensory Intensity," *Behavioral and Brain Sciences* 4 (1981): 175-89, based on data from R.M. Warren, "Elimination of Biases in Loudness Judgements for Tones," *Journal of the Acoustical Society of America* 48 (1970): 1397-1403 and from R. M. Warren "Quantification of Loudness," *American Journal of Psychology* 86 (1973): 807-25.

are shown in figure 4.1. It can be seen that the extent of asymmetric range biases (as measured by deviations from the dashed diagonal line) differed for direct numerical judgments and those derived from marks on the line. But judgments at mid-range with both procedures corresponded to about –6 dB in keeping with PC theory.

Effect of Reverberation on Loudness Functions

Experimental studies of loudness usually employ continuous sounds such as tones and noises. However, many sounds are discontinuous. Speech is an example of a discontinuous complex sound, having both silent pauses and rapid transitions from one speech sound to the next. Reverberation is an important cue to the distance of a speaker, as discussed in chapter 2. If the theory that loudness judgments are based upon distance is valid, reverberation should have an important effect upon the loudness of speech. Normally, as discussed earlier, the ratio of direct to reverberant sound varies with distance, and a convincing illusion of a change in distance of a speaker requires a change in this ratio (see Békésy, 1960; Maxfield, 1931; Steinberg & Snow, 1934). However, loudness experiments normally involve use of an attenuator which alters the overall intensity without varying the ratio of direct to reverberant components. Pollack (1952) found that speech required a greater attenuation for half-loudness judgments than would be expected from the sone scale. Warren, Sersen, and Pores (1958) confirmed Pollack's finding that half-loudness judgments with voice required a greater attenuation than did tone. They used an additional group of subjects who were tested under identical conditions used for the loudness group, except that they were instructed to estimate the effect of doubling distance from the hidden sound source. It was found that estimates of the effect of doubling distance required greater attenuation for voice than for tone, and that half-loudness and twice-distance estimates were equivalent for each type of sound. Warren and his colleagues concluded that the extra attenuation required for voice was necessary to overcome conflict with the unchanging ratio of direct to reverberant sound indicating that the distance to the source of the voice was fixed.

Warren (1973b) manipulated reverberation of speech in a series of loudness experiments using the single judgment procedure described earlier. When the stimulus was a recording of speech with low reverberation (made in an acoustically "dead" radio studio with the microphone close to the speaker's mouth), the intensity change required for half-loudness judgments was about −12 dB as shown by the square symbols in figure 4.2. These results are quite different from those obtained with tone and with noise (see Fig. 4.1), in keeping with earlier reports that greater attenuation was required for half-loudness judgments with speech.

As discussed in chapter 2, listeners can abstract direct from reverberant components, and appear to use these direct components in making some types of localization judgments. But what if direct components were lacking and only reverberant components were present? It is possible to prepare a recording with a high proportion of reverberant sound for which direct components are inaudible. Since only changes in the direct components are correlated with changes in relative distance, listeners should not be able to

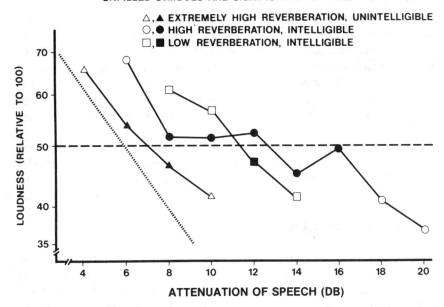

FILLED SYMBOLS ARE NOT SIGNIFICANTLY DIFFERENT FROM 50
UNFILLED SYMBOLS ARE SIGNIFICANTLY DIFFERENT FROM 50

△,▲ EXTREMELY HIGH REVERBERATION, UNINTELLIGIBLE
○,● HIGH REVERBERATION, INTELLIGIBLE
□,■ LOW REVERBERATION, INTELLIGIBLE

LOUDNESS (RELATIVE TO 100)

ATTENUATION OF SPEECH (DB)

Fig. 4.2. The profound effects of reverberation on loudness functions for speech. Numerical judgments of loudness are shown for different attenuations of three 85 dB standards. (Each standard was assigned a loudness value of 100.) The horizontal dashed line represents the mid-range value of 50 free from asymmetrical response bias for monotonic loudness functions, and the diagonal dotted line corresponds to loudness proportional to the square root of the stimulus intensity. Each data point represents the mean of first numerical judgments from a separate group of 30 subjects listening through headphones.

Source: Figure from R.M. Warren, "Measurement of Sensory Intensity," *Behavioral and Brain Sciences* 4 (1981): 175-89; based on data from R. M. Warren, "Anomolous Loudness Function for Speech," *Journal of the Acoustical Society of America* 54 (1973): 390-96.

estimate this physical correlate of loudness with such sounds. Therefore, we should get an anomalous loudness function in which subjective magnitudes would not change in a regular fashion with change in intensity. Warren (1973b) obtained loudness judgments with such highly reverberant (but still intelligible) speech, and the results are summarized by the circular symbols in figure 4.2. As anticipated, an anomalous function was obtained for which loudness did not change with intensity over a wide range of comparison levels. As can be seen in this figure, attenuations from 8 dB through 16 dB were not significantly different from half-loudness for this highly reverberant speech.

In another part of this study, extremely reverberant speech was employed for loudness judgments. This stimulus was prepared through successive recordings each made under highly reverberant conditions. After six such rerecordings, the speech was a completely unintelligible babble, more like noise than speech. As shown by the triangular symbols in figure 4.2, the loudness function obtained with this stimulus resembled the loudness function for Gaussian noise (see Fig. 4.1) more closely than either of the other loudness functions for speech.

To summarize this work with recorded voices, it appears that reverberation is important in determining the loudness of speech, and that manipulation of reverberation produces effects consistent with its role as a cue to distance.

Loudness of Self-Generated Sound

While loudness experiments usually employ subjects operating as sound receivers, subjects can also estimate loudness while operating as sound generators. Loudness experiments based on self-generated sound have some interesting characteristics. The experimenter is not faced with troublesome choices concerning the psychophysical methods to be employed for presenting stimuli to the subject, along with problems concerning possible biases associated with each of these procedures. With self-generated sounds, adjustment of the comparison is done by subjects using their self-contained equipment. It is necessary only to instruct them to produce a sound at a steady level and then at a second steady level, say, one-half that of the first. A number of sounds can be used, and those employed experimentally for loudness judgments have been the periodic sound of a vowel, the noise of a sibilant phoneme, and a nonvocal periodic sound produced by blowing through an instrument producing a tone. The ratio of direct to reverberant sound does not influence judgments of loudness for self-generated sounds, since this ratio does not change with intensity when the subject is the source. Evidence indicates that the same physical correlate (distance) operates for self-generated sounds and for externally generated sounds. When subjects operate as generators, they appear to control intensity (in accordance with the inverse square law) so that target listeners at particular distances can be provided with desired intensity levels; when subjects operate as receivers, they appear to evaluate the intensity of nonreverberant components (in accordance with the inverse square law) in order to determine the distance of the speaker.

An experiment was undertaken to determine whether subjects could adjust the level of different types of self-generated sounds (the vowel "ah," the unvoiced consonant "sh," and a note blown on a pitch pipe) so as to keep the intensity at a target microphone constant for a particular sound when its distance was changed from 10 feet to 5 feet (Warren, 1968a). It was found that mean intensity changes produced to compensate for the effect of this two-fold change in distance varied from 6 to 8 dB with these three sounds, in good agreement with the 6 dB corresponding to the inverse square law. In an earlier experiment with these same three sounds (Warren, 1962), it had been found that an equivalent attenuation (approximately 7 dB) corresponded to half-loudness judgments with each.

The first published study of the loudness of self-generated sounds was that of Lane, Catania, and Stevens (1961). They had used a single sound, "ah," and reported that –6 dB corresponded to half-subjective magnitude. They concluded that "autophonic" judgments of the intensity of self-generated sound yields a power function with an exponent of 0.5. It was also reported that, when masking noise was introduced through headphones while the subject was producing the sound, the same autophonic function was produced. Thus, it appears that nonauditory cues (such as information concerning muscular effort) can substitute for auditory monitoring of sound production, and that such complementary systems for evaluating sound level produce judgments of relative intensity in agreement with each other. However, there is evidence that auditory feedback is necessary for the most delicate control of the intensity of self-generated sounds (Bouhuys, 1966).

Learning of a New Physical Correlate for Loudness

When subjects participate in loudness experiments, they probably are making judgments of a sort never made by them before. That is, they are required to give numerical values to subjective magnitudes. Thus, the physical correlate of loudness reflects the demands of the experimental procedure, and is established on the spot. When subjects have familiarity with another physical scale associated with the level of stimulation, they can use this scale as a physical correlate. For example, subjects familiar with the deciBel scale have been found to use it as the basis for subjective magnitude judgments. Ham and Parkinson (1932) observed that familiarity with deciBel measurements resulted in loudness functions based on this logarithmic scale of sound pressure level. They were forced to abandon the use of subjects having experience with sound measurement and switch to college students without such experience for their formal experiments. A similar problem was described by Laird, Taylor, and Willie (1932), who reported that subjects who were familiar with calibration of audiometers would choose approximately one-half the dB level when asked to judge half-loudness, so that 30 dB was selected as half the loudness of a 60 dB standard. They found that it was not possible for their subjects to ignore their experience with dB levels. Finally,

Rowley and Studebaker (1969) encountered the same difficulty when they used graduate students in audiology as their subjects. Despite repeated attempts to explain that the experimenters were interested in the *subjective* magnitude of loudness rather than the physical level in deciBels, subjects could not give up using the deciBel level as the physical correlate of their loudness judgments.

Perhaps it should be considered that subjects basing loudness judgments upon experience with deciBel levels were not making "errors" in using this scale as the basis for loudness judgments. They had a different physical correlate than those who could not estimate values in deciBels, but such a subjective scale based on measurement of stimulus magnitudes would seem to be at least as valid as one based upon distance.

THE *MEL* SCALE OF PITCH MAGNITUDE

Tones have been characterized not only by the psychological magnitude of loudness, but also by the psychological magnitude of pitch. Stevens, Volkmann, and Newman (1937) constructed the *mel* scale for quantifying the pitch of sinusoidal tones as a function of frequency. Their subjects were instructed to estimate half-pitch for frequencies of a standard ranging from 125 through 12,000 Hz. The results they obtained are summarized in figure 4.3. It can be seen that for the lower end of the range, values of about half-frequency were generally selected as half-pitch (the comparisons chosen for these frequencies averaged about 57 percent). Wever (1949) noted this tendency to choose half-frequency as half-pitch; and stated that, for low tones, the results could be explained as the direct appreciation of frequency differences, so that two intervals of pitch which seemed equal contained the same number of Hertz. However, Wever did not suggest why this simple relation was found.

A clue to the possible basis for the *mel* scale is furnished by Helmholtz's statement that the "...musical scale is as it were the divided rod, by which we measure progressions in pitch, as rhythm measures progression in time." Helmholtz pointed out that the basic unit of musical scales is the octave, and figure 4.3 shows that approximately a one octave drop in frequency corresponded to half-pitch for the lower range of standard frequencies. Why the deviation from this relationship at higher frequencies? The vertical dotted line in the figure shows the upper limit of the musical scale at about 4,500 Hz, and (as described in chapter 3) octaves cannot be estimated accurately for sinusoidal tones above the limits of the musical range (Ward, 1954). Therefore, the octave could not be used as the basis for relative pitch judgments for the three standards above 4,500 Hz. It can be seen in figure 4.3 that, at the highest frequency employed for construction of the *mel* scale (12,000 Hz),

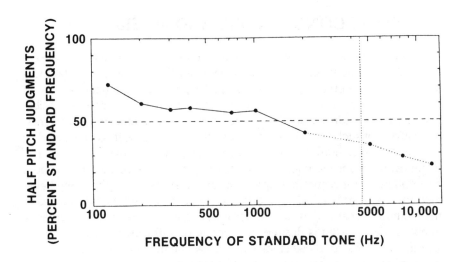

Fig. 4.3. Percent of the standard's frequency selected as half-pitch. The horizontal dashed line corresponding to 50 percent represents frequencies one octave below the standard. The dotted vertical line at 4,500 Hz corresponds to the upper limit of the range of orchestral instruments. The data points lying within the range of orchestral instruments are connected by solid lines; other points are connected by dotted lines.

Source: R.M. Warren, "A Basis for Judgments of Sensory Intensity," *American Journal of Psychology* 71 (1958): 675-87; based on data from S.S. Stevens, J. Volkmann, and E.B. Newman, "A Scale for the Measurement of the Psychological Magnitude Pitch," *Journal of the Acoustical Society of America* 8 (1937): 185-90. Figure copyright 1958 by K.M. Dallenbach, reproduced by permission of the University of Illinois Press.

half-pitch judgments corresponded to a decrease of more than two octaves, so that subjects did not choose a comparison frequency outside the range of musical pitch, even for the highest standard frequencies used.

Stevens, Volkmann, and Newman made an interesting observation concerning the responses of a trained musician who served as one of their subjects, and who gave half-pitch judgments differing from those of the rest of the group. The musician reported that he found that it was very difficult for him to avoid using the octave or some other familiar musical interval in judging half-pitch, and he consciously tried to avoid such settings. However, the musically untrained subjects did not try to avoid the octave, and appeared to base their judgments on this interval for frequencies within the musical pitch range.

SOME CONCLUSIONS AND INFERENCES

If it is accepted that judgments of sensory intensity are disguised estimates of physical magnitudes, can it still be maintained that sensation can be measured directly? Perhaps surprisingly, yes! By defining a loudness scale in terms of a particular set of procedures and calculations, it becomes possible to construct a loudness function on the basis of experimental measurements. The validity of such a scale cannot be questioned because it is established by definition (postulation). However, extreme caution is needed in using operational definitions in psychophysics since more is involved than providing a description of a measurement procedure: the existence of the entity being measured is postulated! Bertrand Russell once described the advantages of the method of postulation as considerable, and equivalent to the advantages of appropriating what is desired over acquiring it through work.

If, as suggested, these studies of "subjective magnitude" deal with estimates of physical magnitudes, it would appear more useful to study directly the bases for estimating physical magnitudes and factors producing errors in judgment. Such an outer-directed psychophysics would further the understanding of how sensory systems are used for appropriate interaction with the environment.

5

Perception of
Acoustic Sequences

Perception of acoustic sequences is of great importance in hearing. Since it is necessary to distinguish between different orders of component sounds in listening to speech and music, it is often assumed that temporal resolution of successive items is required, with a blurring and perceptual inability to distinguish between permuted orders taking place if sounds follow each other too rapidly. However, recent evidence indicates that this common-sense assumption is false. Even when components follow each other at rates too rapid to permit identification of order, changes in their arrangement can be recognized readily. Perception of speech and music seems to involve initial recognition of groupings consisting of several sounds. If required, component sounds and their orders may be inferred for these familiar sequences, even though they cannot be perceived directly.

RATE AT WHICH COMPONENT SOUNDS OCCUR IN SPEECH AND MUSIC

First, let us consider speech as a sequence of phonemes. The sounds composing speech occur at rates of 10 per second or more (average duration of 100 msec or less). Conversational English contains about 120 to 150 words per minute, and since the average word has about 5 phonemes, this results in about 80 to 100 msec per phoneme (Efron, 1963). It should, of course, be kept in mind that individual phonemes vary greatly in duration, and that the boundaries separating temporally contiguous phonemes are often not sharply defined. Oral reading is more rapid than spontaneous speech, and this higher rate of about 170 words per minute corresponds to about 70 msec per phoneme. Joos (1948) stated that at average durations of about 50 msec

119

for phonemes, intelligibility of speech starts to decline. Devices have been developed making it possible to accelerate recorded speech without introducing the pitch change which would result from simply increasing the playback speed, and Foulke and Sticht (1969) have summarized evidence that some comprehension of this "compressed speech" is still possible at rates exceeding 400 words per minute, or an average of about 30 msec per phoneme.

Notes forming melodies usually occur at rates approximating those of syllables in speech rather than those of phonemes. Fraisse (1963) has stated that, while the rate at which notes of a melodic theme are played varies considerably depending upon the composer and the piece (and presumably the performer as well), the fastest rate within the normal range corresponds to about 150 msec per note. However, it appears to be possible to recognize melodies down to about 50 msec per note. While shorter durations have been used by some composers (for example, Liszt and Ravel) the effect produced by such rapid playing is that of a "flickering or rustling" (Winckel, 1967).

Thus, it appears that the average duration of the component sounds forming speech or melodies is greater than 50 msec. Some degree of speech comprehension appears possible when the average duration of phonemes is as low as 30 msec, and some degree of melodic recognition appears possible for notes played at the rate of one each 50 msec.

IDENTIFICATION OF COMPONENTS AND THEIR ORDER

Hirsh (1959) stated that it is necessary to identify phonemes and their orders before words can be recognized. In order to investigate the minimum separation necessary for identification of order, he used pairs of sounds selected from a variety of hisses, tones, and clicks. It was found that differences in onsets of about 20 msec allowed 75 percent correct responses of order with practiced subjects. Hirsh cited the word pair "mitts" and "mist" as an example of word discrimination based upon temporal order identification. Since a hiss resembles the fricative sound /s/, and a click the brief sound bursts of the plosive /t/, he suggested that the ability to distinguish whether a click comes before or after a hiss in his temporal resolution experiments was an "experimental analog" of the "mitts"/"mist" distinction.

Following Hirsh's experiment, Broadbent and Ladefoged (1959) used pairs of sounds selected from hiss, buzz, and pip (tone). They found that individuals at first could not name the order of successive sounds each lasting 150 msec, but after some experience with the task the order could be named accurately at 30 msec durations (approximating the value reported earlier by Hirsh for practiced observers). Broadbent and Ladefoged commented that temporal ordering seemed to be made on the basis of "quality" rather than "...a difference of a type normally described as a difference in perceived order." (We shall return to this comment concerning sound quality when we describe the distinction between pattern recognition and the naming of order.)

Hirsh and Sherrick (1961) employed bings (pulses sent through a circuit resonant at 666 Hz) and bongs (like bings, but the circuit was resonant at 278 Hz). These sounds were described as resembling xylophone notes of high and low pitch. In one experiment, they found that when the bings and bongs were delivered sequentially to the same ear (conditions similar to the earlier studies of Hirsh and of Ladefoged and Broadbent), discrimination of order was possible down to about 20 msec temporal separation with trained subjects. They also had the bing delivered to one ear and the bong to the other (the threshold for discriminating order was again about 20 msec), and only one sound (the bing) delivered to separate ears successively (threshold for discriminating which ear received the first sound once more was about 20 msec). Hirsh and Sherrick also reported that the thresholds for perception of order for pairs of successive stimuli were approximately the same whether the two events were light flashes in different parts of the visual field, two vibrations (one to each hand), or two different types of stimuli one to each of two sensory modalities. They concluded that the value of 20 msec is a fundamental limit for perception of order, which is independent of the modality employed.

Values close to those reported by Hirsh for temporal resolution of pairs of nonspeech sounds have been reported by other laboratories. Both Kinney (1961) and Fay (1966) found that resolution was possible at about 30 msec separation. Fay commented that, since both Kinney's and his experiments employed "untrained" subjects, practice could well result in improvement to the 20 msec value of Hirsh (1959).

Fay also used pairs of recorded sustained speech sounds, and found that his unpracticed subjects could identify the order for some phoneme pairs with excellent resolution (e.g., 10 msec for /v/ and /1/), while other phoneme pairs were even more difficult to resolve than pairs of tones (e.g., /m/ and /n/ could not be ordered at onset disparities of 70 msec).

Efron (1963) reasoned that aphasias might be associated with a general difficulty in ordering sound. He used subjects having brain damage associated with language impairment. It was found that the temporal separation of 10 msec tones (2,500 Hz "bleep" and 250 Hz "bop") required for perception of order was very much greater for receptive aphasic patients (who could speak but not understand when spoken to) than for either normal controls or expressive aphasic patients (who could understand speech, but could not themselves speak properly). Tallal and Piercy (1973, 1974) using pairs of sounds, and Brookshire (1972) and Bond (1976) employing recycled sequences of four different sounds (the rationale for using recycled sequences will be discussed later), also found that aphasics and dysphasics exhibited poorer performance than did normal controls in tasks requiring identification of temporal order. Carmon and Nachshon (1971) used recycled four-item sequences and compared patients with unilateral lesions of right and left hemispheres with control subjects free from neurological disorders. They found that patients with lesions of the left hemisphere (the dominant hemisphere subserving speech) differed from both of the other groups. The investigators in all of these studies of aphasia assumed that the ability to distinguish the order of sounds was necessary for the perception of speech, and that the impairment of this ability was one of the possible causes of aphasias and dysphasias. However, this is not the only interpretation. As we shall see, there is reason to believe that identification of temporal order cannot be accomplished without verbal labeling of stimuli within a sequence, so that poor performance could be a consequence rather than a cause of aphasia.

TEMPORAL ORDER IDENTIFICATION WITHIN EXTENDED SEQUENCES

While reports based upon pairs of sounds in the 1950s and 1960s had indicated an ability to identify order down to a lower limit of temporal separation of about 20 to 50 msec, there were a few observations in the 1950s indicating that some complex sequences required much longer separation times for identification of order. Heise and Miller (1951) reported that, when a sequence of several tones each lasting 125 msec had one member which differed greatly from the frequency of the other components, it would "pop out" of the ordered group so that listeners could not tell which sounds were temporally contiguous with it. There also was a report by Ladefoged (1959), which was later described in more detail by Ladefoged and Broadbent (1960), that the locations of clicks or other extraneous sounds in sentences are grossly mislocalized, listeners sometimes reporting the occurrences a word or two away from their actual locations. These difficulties in perceiving order were considered to represent an interference in normal ordering ability caused by special attentional and information processing mechanisms associated with speech and music.

However, there is a quite different way of interpreting these examples of an inability to identify order. Recent experiments have suggested that the naming of the order of components within extended sequences having item durations as brief as the sounds of speech rests upon the initial recognition of groupings or larger patterns, from which individual constituents and their arrangements can be inferred. This theory concerning identification of order was developed as a consequence of experiments using repeated or recycled sequences.

Recycled sequences have been used to study the ability to perceive the order of successive sounds since they permit a limited number of sounds (usually three or four) to be used to produce relatively simple stimuli of indefinite duration. Recycled sequences can be prepared by recording statements of each of the desired sounds, cutting segments of the tapes corresponding to the desired durations, and splicing these segments into a loop which can play the same order over and over. However, these sequences also may be generated directly ("on line") using signal sources in conjunction with programming equipment. Recycled sequences of two sounds represent simple alternation with only one possible arrangement, sequences of three sounds have two possible arrangements, and four sounds have six possible arrangements (a sequence of n sounds has factorial [n − 1] arrangements). Experimenters usually allow listeners to listen as long as they wish, and to name the order starting with whichever sound they choose while the sequence continues to be heard. Although the first and last sounds of a sequence can be identified easily (Warren, 1972), identification of the sound present when a recycled sequence is turned on does not help in determining the relative order of components, and there is no last sound since subjects respond before termination of the sequence.

Identification of Order for Sequences of Unrelated Sounds and for Sequences of Speech Sounds

The first study to use recycled sequences reported a surprising inability of listeners to identify the order of components (Warren, 1968b; see also Warren, Obusek, Farmer, & Warren, 1969). Listeners heard a sequence of four sounds consisting of successive steady statements of a hiss, a tone, a buzz, and the speech sound "ee." Each item lasted 200 msec, and the sounds were played over and over in the same order. It was found that the listeners could not name the temporal arrangement even though the duration was well above the classical limit for detection of order. Although it was possible to identify each of the sounds, the order remained frustratingly elusive. In another part of the initial study, a recycled sequence was employed consisting of four spoken digits (one, three, eight, two, one, three,...), each complete statement of the four numbers taking 800 msec. In order to avoid any transitional cues to order, each digit was recorded separately. Despite the fact that each of the words was itself complex, so that presumably phonemic orders had to be established within each digit, correct identification was accomplished with ease by all listeners.

The final part of the initial study dealt with the identification of temporal order for recycled sequences of four vowels. A 200 msec segment was cut from a tape recording of an extended steady statement of each vowel. These were spliced together to form a loop of tape which repeated the vowels without transitions or pauses between sounds. (Of course, a person could not produce such abrupt changes while speaking.) Although it was fairly difficult to judge the order, the performance of subjects was significantly above chance. The task became considerably easier when each of these vowels was reduced to 150 msec with 50 msec of silence separating items; and it was easiest of all with single complete statements of vowels each possessing natural onset and decay characteristics. (Again, each vowel lasted about 150 msec with 50 msec silences without transitional cues linking successive phonemes.) Subsequent work by Thomas, Hill, Carroll, and Garcia (1970) and by Thomas, Cetti, and Chase (1971) indicated that the threshold for naming order within a recycled sequence of four concatenated steady-state vowels was 125 msec, with the threshold dropping to 100 msec when brief silent intervals were inserted beween the steady-state vowels. Cole and Scott (1973) and Dorman, Cutting, and Raphael (1975) found that introduction of normal articulatory transitions linking successive items facilitated identification of order with recycled phonemic sequences. And finally, Cullinan, Erdos, Schaefer, and Tekieli (1977) used recycled sequences consisting of a variety of vowels and consonant-vowel syllables, and concluded that lower thresholds were associated with a greater resemblance of the phonetic sequences to those occurring in normal speech.

Thus, it appears that the identification of order within sequences of speech sounds is a rather special process facilitated by articulatory transitions between phonemes of the sort normally encountered within speech. Possible mechanisms underlying our ability to name phonemic orders will be discussed subsequently.

Identification of Order within Tonal Sequences

Successive tones of different frequencies form sequences having special interest for two reasons: (1) it is possible to control the extent of frequency differences between sounds so that the items can be made nearly identical or very different; (2) tonal sequences are related to melodic perception and music.

It is known that perceptual splitting of a pair of interleaved melodies can occur when each is played in a separate register. Two separate melodies can be heard under these conditions as a result of the domination of pitch contiguity over temporal contiguity (Ortmann, 1926). Interleaving of melodic lines has been used by Baroque composers, such as Bach and Telemann, so that a single instrument can seem to produce two simultaneous melodies. This melodic segregation has been called "implied polyphony" by Bukofzer (1947) and "compound melodic line" by Piston (1947), each of whom gave examples of its use in Baroque compositions. Dowling (1973) has named this separation "melodic fission." A demonstration of the separation of simultaneous melodies was given at a meeting in Teddington, England, by Warren (1968b) who played a piano recording of Professor Gregoria Suchy playing "God Save the Queen" and "America the Beautiful" with the notes from each melody alternated. Neither of the interleaved melodies could be recognized when both were played in the same register, even with instructions to try to link together alternate notes. But when the notes of each melody were played in different registers, it was easy to recognize each. It was suggested at the time that simultaneous conversations as well as simultaneous melodies can form "parallel auditory continua" which remain perceptually separated without temporal cross-linking.

A separation process which was called "primary auditory stream segregation" was reported by Bregman and Campbell (1971) for recycled sequences of six tones, three in a cluster of low and three in a cluster of high frequencies. They stated that it appeared to be easier to identify order within as opposed to across clusters. Thomas and Fitzgibbons (1971) reported that successive tones within recycled sequences of four items all have to be within half an octave for accurate identification of order at the limiting value of 125 msec per item. However, a decrease in accuracy of identifying order within increasing frequency separation was not found in subsequent studies involving recycled sequences of four tones by Nickerson and Freeman (1974) and Warren and Byrnes (1975). While there can be little doubt that splitting into parallel auditory streams occurs in Baroque compositions having "compound melodic lines," it appears to be rather difficult to obtain analogous splitting with nonmelodic recycled tonal sequences.

Before dealing further with the important problem of perception of sequences of sounds which are all within the same continuum or stream as in speech or musical melodies, let us return to the great difficulty in identifying the order within extended sequences of unrelated sounds. An early hypothesis by Bregman and Campbell (1971) considered that each of the sounds in recycled sequences of four unrelated items formed a separate auditory stream with its own repetition, resulting in perceptual equivalence of permuted orders. However, as we shall see, subsequent experiments have shown that different arrangements of items within such sequences form readily distinguishable patterns, so that permuted orders are not perceptually equivalent. It is only the *naming* of the order of components that requires long item durations, and recent evidence has indicated that the rate-determining stage in identification of order is the time required for providing verbal labels for the sounds.

Identification of Order and Verbal Labeling

Of course, it is possible to name the order of items within recycled sequences if their durations are sufficiently long. For example, if a repeated sequence consisting of hisses, tones, and buzzes is heard with each sound lasting one second, virtually everyone can call out the correct order. This achievement hardly seems surprising since listeners can name each sound as it occurs. But when groups of untrained subjects were allowed to listen to sequences of unrelated sounds for as long as they wished before calling out the order, the threshold for performance significantly better than chance was between 450 and 670 msec per item for recycled four-item sequences. This threshold fell to between 200 and 300 msec when different groups of subjects responded by arranging cards bearing the names of the four items in the order of occurrence (Warren & Obusek, 1972). Card-ordering permitted listeners to break the task into parts by listening for one sound, and then trying to identify the sound immediately preceding or following. The task of identifying order can be made somewhat easier by using recycled sequences consisting of three different sounds (for which there are only two possible arrangements). With three-item sequences, subjects can choose one of the sounds as an anchor, and make a single decision concerning which of the remaining two components follows this sound. The problem is then completely solved; the remaining sound must precede the anchor. Using this procedure with an unlimited time for responding and cards to facilitate the task, the threshold was found to be about 200 msec per item with untrained subjects (Warren & Ackroff, 1976a).

Why does the lower limit for identification of order occur at approximately 200 msec per item? A clue to a possible answer is furnished by the observation of Helmholtz (1887) and Garner (1951) that the number of identical acoustic events within extended sequences cannot be counted at rates above five or six items per second.

Both counting and naming of the order of items consist of the attaching of distinctive verbal labels to successive events. It has been suggested that it is the time required for verbal labeling of an ongoing stimulus that sets the limiting rate of item presentation, not only for counting, but for the naming of order within sequences of sounds (Warren, 1974a). Successful performances for both of these tasks was considered to require that the verbal encoding of one item be completed before the onset of the next.

Short sequences may not require labeling of each item as it occurs. It was found by Garner (1951) that low numbers of identical tone-bursts (up to about four to six) could be counted at twice the presentation rate required for

higher numbers of tone-bursts; and Warren (1972) reported that the introduction of three seconds of silence between repetitions of sequences containing three or four unrelated sounds, each of 200 msec duration, made it
possible for the order of items to be named accurately. Perhaps both counting and ordering can be accomplished after termination of a short sequence if
labeling of the successive items can be completed before the short-duration
memory trace fades. Assuming that the maximum readout speed from
storage corresponds to the maximum speed of verbal labeling observed for
the numbering of extended sequences or for the naming of unrelated sounds
(roughly 200 msec per item), the storage time between termination of a sound
and completion of its verbal encoding need be no more than about one
second for the four- to six-item sequences used by Garner (1951) or the three-
or four-item sequences used by Warren (1972). This time limit for readout of
stored auditory images is within the limits of one or two seconds observed
with other tasks. [See Neisser (1967) on "echoic storage"; Norman (1967) on
"tape-recorder memory."] Additional help in naming order with short
sequences is given by the ease with which initial and terminal sounds can be
identified (Warren, 1972).

Recycled sequences consisting of vowels and of monosyllabic words are
especially interesting. Rapid verbal encoding would be anticipated since not
only are the listeners very familiar with these sounds but, perhaps more
importantly, the sound is the name: that is, the names of the sounds, and the
sounds of the names, are the same.

As noted earlier, recycled sequences consisting of four vowels can be
ordered, under optimal conditions, at a presentation rate of about 100 msec
per item (Dorman, Cutting, & Raphael, 1975; Thomas, Cetti, & Chase, 1971).
The relative ease of identifying order when the verbal label and the stimulus
are identical is not restricted to sequences of single phonemes. Warren
(1968b) and Warren and Warren (1970) reported that, when each of four
items in an iterated sequence consisted of a word (a digit), naming of order
was at least as easy with four recycled vowels, and a "personal observation"
of Yntema and Norman (cited by Norman, 1967) indicated that noniterated
sequences of digits could be identified with some degree of accuracy at 100
msec per digit.

Teranishi (1977) measured the minimum item durations permitting the
identification of order within various four-item recycled sequences consisting
of either nonrelated sounds or Japanese vowels. He independently arrived at
the same explanation proposed by Warren (1974a): that is, the time required
for naming component sounds is the rate-determining step in the identification of order, and that the order of sequences of vowels can be identified at
high presentation rates because the sounds themselves are verbal labels.

If verbal encoding time sets the limit for naming of order within auditory
sequences, we would expect similar limits set by verbal encoding time for

visual sequences. Terence O'Brien and Anne Treisman in 1970 determined the threshold for discrimination of order for three visual items, such as successive geometrical figures or successive colors, when recycled in a three-channel tachistoscope (personal communication). They found the same threshold which has been reported for recycled three-item auditory sequences of nonrelated sounds: that is, 200 msec per item. Sperling and Reeves (1980) presented a rapid string of digits on a cathode-ray tube and reported that, although their subjects could perceive the digits, they could not tell their order. They stated that this difficulty was "analogous" to that described by Warren for sequences of sounds.

The discussion thus far has dealt with the importance of verbal encoding for perception of temporal order. Other experiments dealing with the topic of memory have indicated that while recall of events does not require verbal encoding, recall of the order of events does.

Need for Verbal Labeling for Serial Order Retention in Memory Experiments

There have been several studies in the field of memory dealing with verbal encoding and the accuracy of recalling the serial order of sequential items. Paivio and Csapo (1969) presented sequences consisting of printed words or pictures of familiar objects. When the presentation rate was too rapid to permit naming of pictured items (but not the printed words), the pictures could be recalled as accurately as the words, but only the word sequences permitted retention of order information. When the presentation rate was slowed so that the objects in the pictures could be named, tasks requiring temporal ordering of the pictures could be handled readily. Del Castillo and Gumenik (1972) used drawings of objects and found that the "nameability" of depicted objects and the presentation rate both influenced recall of order in a manner consistent with the hypothesis that accurate ordering by subjects requires naming of items at the time of presentation. Similar observations were made by Philipchalk and Rowe (1971) who compared recall of order for sequences consisting of familiar sounds with recall of order for sequences consisting of words, and found that performance was poorer for the sequences of nonverbal sounds. Finally, Rowe and Cake (1977) used a variety of presentation rates and compared ordered recall for sequences of sounds, and sequences of the verbal labels for these same sounds. They found that, for their seven-item sequences, performance was poorer for the sounds than for the words at interstimulus intervals of 500 msec, with this difference disappearing at interstimulus intervals of one second. They extended their study to serial probe, probe recognition, and running memory span, and found the words superior to the sounds in the recency component of the serial position curve in all cases. They concluded that their results supported the theory that verbal encoding facilitates ordering and conflicted with explanations based on higher-order processing strategies or retrieval problems. These results are consistent with Paivio's (1971) two-process theory of memory (which emphasizes differences between verbal and nonverbal encoding of information), as well as with the hypothesis that the rate-limiting process for identification of order with recycled sequences of nonverbal sounds involves the verbal encoding time for individual components.

IDENTIFICATION OF PATTERNS WITHOUT DISCRIMINATION OF ORDER: HOLISTIC PATTERN RECOGNITION

In the 1970s, evidence became available indicating that it was possible to discriminate between permuted orders of two brief sounds well below the limit of 20 msec cited by Hirsh (1959) for the naming of order. Patterson and Green (1970) used pairs of brief click-like sounds called Huffman sequences which have identical power spectra but different phase spectra, so that the only difference between members of a pair is in the temporal arrangement. They found that Huffman sequences permitted discrimination between temporal orders down to 2.5 msec. Yund and Efron (1974) found that listeners could discriminate between permuted orders of a two-item sequence (such as two tones of different frequencies) down to temporal separations of only one or two msec. Efron (1973) emphasized that such "micropatterns" were perceived as unitary perceptual events, with different qualities associated with the different orders. Listeners could not identify the order of components within these brief sequences unless information was provided to them. However, once they had learned the temporal order corresponding to the characteristic quality of the stimulus pair, they could "infer" the correct order on subsequent presentation. Wier and Green (1975) subsequently reported "nearly perfect" discrimination between the permuted orders of sequences of two tones having a total duration of two msec.

The ability to discriminate between permuted arrangements of sounds at durations well below the limit permitting unaided identification of order also has been reported for recycled sequences. Wilcox, Neisser, and Roberts (1972) first reported that trained listeners could tell whether pairs of recycled sequences containing four items had the same or permuted orders at durations of 100 msec per item, with Warren (1972) subsequently reporting similar results for untrained listeners.

The extent of training can have a profound effect upon the detection of differences between complex sequences. Watson and his colleagues (Watson, 1976; Watson, Wroton, Kelly, & Benbassat, 1975; Watson, Kelly, & Wroton, 1976) have studied the effects of training upon the discrimination of tonal sequences designed to have a temporal complexity and frequency range comparable to those of spoken words. In a typical experiment, "word length" sequences consisting of ten 40 msec tones were used, and the effects of training were measured for tasks involving detectability of changes in frequency, intensity, or duration of one component within the sequence. Usually, many hours of training were required to reach asymptotic performance with these ten-item tonal sequences.

Using simpler stimuli (recycled and nonrecycled sequences consisting of three different types of sound), Warren (1974a) found that it was not only quite easy to teach subjects to discriminate between permuted orders down to 5 msec per item, but also that it was easy to teach them the names and order of components within these sequences. Further, as we shall see, learning the names and arrangements of components within sequences consisting of very brief items could take place inadvertently if subjects had practice with the same sequences at longer item durations.

In one experiment within this study, subjects heard pairs of recycled three-item sequences (2,500 Hz sine wave, 1,000 Hz square wave, white noise) with members of each pair consisting of the same items which were arranged either in identical or permuted order. After little training, subjects were able to achieve nearly perfect performance at all item durations (5 through 400 msec). While subjects were able to name order without training at the longest item duration, at the shorter durations (30 msec per item and below), listeners could not even identify the component sounds directly, much less distinguish their order. When asked how they discriminated between the permuted orders of the briefest sounds, none of the listeners mentioned a resolution into component items, and all answers referred to some overall quality, such as "One sounds more like a cricket." Another experiment in this study used nonrecycled two-item and four-item sequences, and attempted to teach listeners to name the order of permuted arrangements at brief item durations with both types of sequences. Following training, the items and their orders could be named accurately at durations down to 10 msec per item. Of course, the naming of order was not a direct identification of components and their orders but, rather, a rote response of a taught verbal label—an incorrect identification of order could have been learned just as easily.

It was pointed out that inadvertent learning of verbal labels could occur in some experiments designed to measure thresholds for identification of order. This training occurs when listeners, presented first with long-item durations for which unaided naming of order is possible, are then presented with a series of sequences having decreasing item durations. We have seen that different arrangements of items are distinguishable at brief item durations, and since sequences differing slightly in durations of components (up to item duration ratios of 1:2) may be recognized as having the same or different orders, the verbal description of the order of the longer sequence may be identified with and transferred to the shorter. Through a series of successive transfers to ever shorter items, a level can be reached which is well below the threshold possible without training. Using this procedure for threshold training, it was possible to obtain correct identification of order in recycled three-item sequences down to ten msec per item without communicating information concerning order to the subjects in any direct fashion (Warren, 1974a).

Extent of Temporal Mismatch Permitting Holistic Pattern Recognition

An experiment was undertaken to determine the extent of mismatch of item durations required to prevent recognition of identical orders within recycled four-item sequences of the same sounds (Warren, 1974b). In order to avoid inadvertent learning of order-equivalence at different item durations, groups of college students were used having no prior experience with experiments dealing with sequences. Subjects were presented with one recycled sequence consisting of tone, noise, extended vowel "ee," and buzz, and a second sequence consisting of either the identical order of the same items or the same items with the order of noise and buzz interchanged. The first sequence always had item durations of 200 msec, and the second sequence had item durations ranging from 127 through 600 msec, as shown in figure 5.l. Separate groups of 30 subjects were used for each of the eight durations of the second sequence, and each subject made only two judgments: one same/different order judgment involving identical arrangement of components, and one same/different order judgment involving permuted arrangement of components (total of 60 judgments obtained for each duration of the second stimulus). The results are shown in figure 5.1. It can be seen that the accuracy of judgments was highest at 200 and 215 msec item durations of the second sequence, and that accuracy decreased monotonically below 200 msec and above 215 msec item durations. The decrease in accuracy at longer item durations is of interest, since direct naming of order became possible at the longest item durations. However, since one of the sequences always had items lasting 200 msec, order could not be identified for this sequence, so that knowledge of the order of the other would be of no help in deciding whether the sequences had same or different arrangements. It was concluded that judgments involved a "temporal template" with the extent of permissible mismatch in durations shown in the figure.

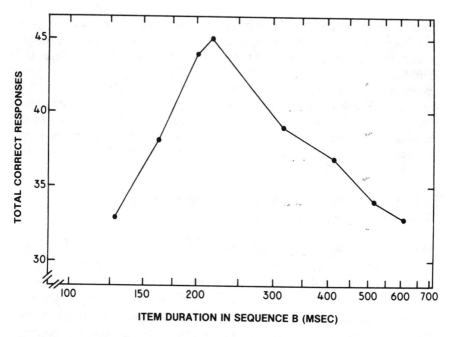

Fig. 5.1. Holistic pattern recognition with temporal mismatch. Scores for correct same-or-different judgments are shown for pairs of recycled sequences consisting of the same four sounds arranged in either identical or permuted orders. Sequence A of the pair always had component sounds lasting 200 msec, and the duration of items in Sequence B is given by the abscissa. The maximum score for correct responses is 60. Each data point is based on the responses of separate groups of 30 subjects.

Source: From R.M. Warren, "Auditory Pattern Discrimination by Untrained Listeners," *Perception & Psychophysics* 15 (1974): 495-500.

Should Trained or Untrained Subjects Be Used?

The question of whether to use trained or untrained subjects in perceptual experiments is an important one since it can have profound effects upon the results obtained. Trained subjects can give much more sensitive responses and make distinctions not possible for untrained subjects. On the other hand, we have seen how subjects can inadvertently be trained to provide correct rote naming of temporal order of sounds lasting only a few milliseconds, even when this information is not provided directly. The report by Divenyi and Hirsh (1974) that highly trained subjects could "identify" the temporal order of nonrecycled three-item tonal sequences at item durations as low as two msec, as well as the report by Neisser and Hirst (1974) that one of their highly trained subjects had a threshold for "identification" of order within recycled and nonrecycled four-item sequences of about 30 msec per component could well represent examples of the results of such rote learning.

The dangers of misinterpreting results attributable to training procedures are not limited to perception of sequences, and have been discussed earlier in relation to other studies such as time-intensity trading, and loudness judgments.

A Comparison of Holistic Pattern Recognition with Identification of Components and Their Orders Using Untrained Subjects

Results described thus far with recycled sequences have suggested that direct naming of the order of components is a fundamentally different task than the recognition of sequences with particular orders, so that distinguishing between permuted orders can take place at item durations much too brief to allow identification of components and their orders. In order to test the validity of these suggestions, 22 separate groups of 30 subjects each heard three-item recycled sequences through headphones and were required either to report the order of components by arranging cards bearing the names of sounds in order of their occurrence, or to report whether two recycled sequences of three components with either identical or permuted orders sounded the same or different (Warren & Ackroff, 1976a).

There were two sets of sounds used for constructing the three-item sequences and, as we shall see, the choice of constituent sounds had a profound effect on same/different judgments, but not upon naming of order. One set consisted of two periodic sounds (2,500 Hz tone and 1,000 Hz square wave), and broad-band noise. The other set consisted of one periodic sound (2,000 Hz tone) and two noises—high-band noise (1/3-octave band centered on 5,000 Hz), and low-band noise (500-1,000 Hz).

Experiment I of this study dealt with the identification of the order of components. After familiarization with the names of the sounds when heard alone, listeners were presented with one recycled three-item sequence and attempted to arrange cards with the names of each sound in the order of occurrence. Following this single judgment, the subjects were dismissed and served in no further sequence experiments. The results obtained are shown in figure 5.2. It can be seen that accuracy of identification of order was significantly above chance for 200 and 400 msec per item, and at chance level for 100 msec per item with both types of sequences.

Experiment II used the same sequences employed in Experiment I, but subjects were not required to identify order. They listened to a pair of sequences containing the same three sounds arranged in identical or per-

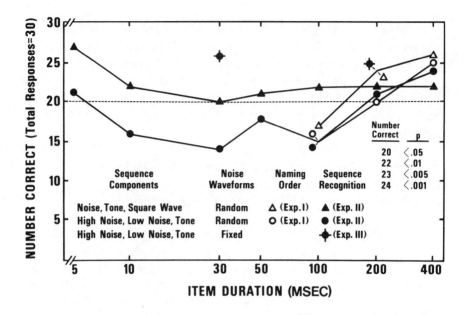

Fig. 5.2. Accuracy of naming the order of components and accuracy of sequence recognition (reporting whether two sequences with the same components had identical or permuted orders) for three-item recycled sequences. On-line generation of random noise bursts was used in Experiment I (naming) and Experiment II (recognition). "Frozen" or fixed waveform noise bursts were used for recognition in Experiment III. The dashed horizontal line corresponds to the limit of performance significantly better than chance.
Source: From R.M. Warren and J.M. Ackroff, "Two Types of Auditory Sequence Perception," *Perception & Psychophysics* 20 (1976): 387-94.

muted orders, and were required to decide whether the two sequences were the same or different. Each subject made two same/different judgments, one involving identical and one involving permuted orders. The results shown in figure 5.2 indicate that, with one noise and two periodic sounds (square wave and tone), performance was significantly above chance at all item durations from 5 through 400 msec. At the shortest item duration of 5 msec, the entire sequence had a period of 15 msec, and a repetition frequency lying in the tonal range (67 Hz), so that the increase in accuracy at this duration might be a consequence of differences in pitch quality of the two arrangements. The results obtained with sequences consisting of one noise and two periodic sounds demonstrates that listeners without any prior training or practice could discriminate between permuted orders down to 5 msec as had been reported earlier for highly trained psychoacoustically sophisticated subjects (Warren, 1974a).

However, the results obtained for same/different judgments with the groups receiving high-band noise, low-band noise, and tone are quite different. It can be seen that judgments were at chance level from 10 through 100 msec per item. At 200 and 400 msec per item, judgments were above chance, but since it had been shown in Experiment I that subjects could identify order at these item durations, same/different judgments could have been mediated by identification of components and their order. The inability to distinguish between permuted orders with item durations in the range of 10 to 100 msec when only one of the components was a periodic sound suggested that successive noise bursts of the same band-pass characteristics might each be treated as a different sound. Although successive bursts of noise derived from the same generators and spectral filters conventionally are treated as samples of the same sound in experiments dealing with sequence perception (Broadbent & Ladefoged, 1959; Fay, 1966; Hirsh, 1959; Neisser & Hirst, 1974; Warren, Obusek, Farmer, & Warren, 1969), the waveform and short-term running spectra are quite different for separate bursts. Thus, sequences consisting of high-band noise, low-band noise, and tone contain only a single periodic sound (the tone) surrounded by ever-changing waveforms. However, when only one of the three items was derived from on-line noise in the sequence consisting of noise, tone, and square wave, the relative positions of the periodic components consisting of tone and square wave could permit listeners to distinguish between the fixed patterns corresponding to the permuted orders, even if the noise did not enter into the judgments.

An experiment was undertaken using the three-item sequences consisting of the tone and two noise bands to test whether differences in successive waveforms of the "same" on-line noise band were responsible for the inability to make same/different judgments. New groups of subjects were presented with iterated sequences containing "frozen" or fixed-waveform noise bursts. By using a digital delay line for repeating segments of the filtered noise bursts together with appropriate programming equipment, listeners heard sequences having unchanging or frozen noise segments for the high-band noise and for the low-band noise, respectively, within each of the two sequences to be compared, whether they were in the same or different item orders. The results shown as Experiment III in figure 5.2 indicate that accuracy increased dramatically with the use of frozen noise segments, so that performance at 30 msec per item was appreciably better with sequences containing two frozen noise bursts than with the sequence consisting of square wave, tone, and broad-band noise. However, frozen waveforms were not required for naming the order of components at long-item durations; the score obtained with frozen waveforms was similar to that obtained with on-line noise bands for sequences with 200 msec items. Other groups of subjects, not shown in the figure, received the same order of components for sequences consisting of high-band noise/low-band noise/tone, but different frozen waveforms for each sequence (that is, each member of the pair of sequences had its own frozen waveforms for the high-band noise and for the low-band noise). When item durations were 30 msec, it was found that subjects considered these sequences having the same nominal order of components but different waveforms to be different.

Holistic Pattern Recognition and Detection of Acoustic Repetition

It is possible to consider a recycled sequence as a periodic sound (see chapter 3). Repeated three-item sequences with periods less than 50 msec have repetition frequencies greater than 20 Hz, and would be expected to generate a pitch corresponding to their particular frequency. Permuted orders would produce the same power spectra, but they could be distinguished on the basis of their different phase spectra. Periods longer than 50 msec correspond to infratonal repetition frequencies, and it has been shown that recognition of infratonal repetition does not require that the iterated pattern contain identifiable component sounds (see Fig. 3.12). However, when individual components exceed a few hundred msec in duration, direct identification of components and their order within a sequence can contribute to pattern identification, so that a holistic pattern recognition is not required.

Holistic Pattern Recognition and Context-Sensitive Speech Sounds

Wickelgren (1969) proposed that identification of the temporal order of phonemes does not occur directly, and that a distinctive perceptual organization occurs from which the order within sequences of phonetic items can be inferred. The distinctive organizations in Wickelgren's model reflect the fact that processes involved in the articulation of adjacent speech sounds can interact and influence each other's acoustic forms. Context-sensitive phonemes (or allophones) can convey usable information concerning the identity of preceding and following speech sounds so that, by recognizing the particular allophonic form of a phoneme, we may identify neighboring phonemes as well. The somewhat different model proposed by Warren (1974a) on the basis of experiments with nonlinguistic sequences considers that the identification of order within sequences of brief sounds involves two stages: recognition of the overall pattern, followed by recitation of the learned multi-element name describing the components and their order. Since it has been shown that the influence of one sound upon the acoustic form of another is not necessary for recognition of patterns of arbitrarily selected sounds having durations equivalent to or briefer than those of phonemes (Warren, 1974a), context sensitivity does not appear to be necessary for recognition of linguistic sequences.

However, allophonic variation might facilitate accurate identification of strings of linguistic sounds under noisy conditions.

Identification of Components and Their Orders and Holistic Pattern Recognition for Dichotomous Patterns

Garner and his associates (Garner & Gottwald, 1967, 1968; Preusser, 1972; Royer & Garner, 1970) used extended patterns consisting of two elements (for example, high tone, low tone). They observed that: 1) the nature of perceptual organization used by subjects changed with item durations; 2) that a recognition task gave different results than an identification task; and 3) some sequences were perceived holistically, without direct identification of the component items. Despite the differences in the extended dichotomous sequences and recycled sequences consisting of three or more sounds, the observations and conclusions derived from experiments with these two types of patterns are similar.

Holistic Pattern Recognition in Animals Other than Humans

It appears that, while animals other than humans can discriminate between permuted orders of sounds within sequences on the basis of a holistic pattern recognition, they are unable to make discriminations based upon identification of components and their order.

Identification of components and their order seems to be possible only for humans since only we appear to have the requisite ability to code, store, and retrieve symbols representing individual sounds. The inability of monkeys to achieve performance characteristic of human identification of sounds and their orders is demonstrated by an experiment by Dewson and Cowey (1969). After considerable training, their three monkeys were able to discriminate accurately between two-item sequences in which each of the items could be either a tone or a noise (there were four possible patterns consisting of tone-tone, noise-noise, tone-noise, and noise-tone) if, and only if, item durations were briefer than approximately 1.5 seconds. When durations were increased to more than three seconds, the monkeys could not master the discrimination, apparently being unable to recall the first item after termination of the second (responses could not be made until termination of the entire sequence). Humans can, of course, easily discriminate between such sequences consisting of three-second items (or, indeed, much longer item durations). But for us, as for monkeys, the actual memory trace of the first sound has probably faded into oblivion within a few seconds, so that the image of the sound itself is not available for discrimination. It is, rather, the *name* of the first sound which persists for us, and which, together with the name of the second sound, provides the basis for discrimination.

It might be argued that monkeys are creatures relying primarily on vision, so that auditory tasks are difficult for these animals. However, this argument would not apply to dolphins. These creatures are readily trainable, and rely upon hearing to a great extent for feeding and for social interaction. Nevertheless, an upper limit for sequence discrimination for the dolphin was reported by Thompson (1976) matching that reported earlier for the monkey. Thompson used four sounds, which can be called, A, B, C, and D, that were used to form two-item sequences. The dolphin was trained to press one paddle for either sequence AC or BD and a different paddle for either sequence AD or BC. The animal was not allowed to respond until the sequence was completed. Thompson stated that increasing the delay interval between the two sounds of the sequence beyond two to three seconds resulted in an abrupt loss in the ability to discriminate between sequences. After using a variety of testing procedures, he concluded that "...it can be ...argued that the 2- to 3- sec ISI (interstimulus interval) delay limit represents a perceptual threshold beyond which the 'wholeness' or gestalt of the configure (sic) is no longer perceived, the animal now hearing two discrete sounds..." (p. 116). Colavita, Szeligo, and Zimmer (1974) trained cats to discriminate between sequences consisting of tonal intensity changes (loud-soft-loud vs. soft-loud-soft), each intensity level lasting 900 msec with 100 msec between levels. As a result of the nature of changes in performance and the ability to relearn following bilateral insular-temporal lesions, these investigators concluded that the cats' original sequence discrimination was holistic, and not based upon pair-wise discrimination of the order of individual intensities. Holistic pattern recognition, it seems, is used by several species of animals to discriminate between permuted orders of brief items.

CONCLUSIONS

It has been assumed for some time that the ability to distinguish between different arrangements of the same sounds requires that listeners be able to identify the order of components. However, recent evidence indicates that permuted orders of speech sounds and permuted orders of unrelated sounds (such as hisses, tones, and buzzes) can be distinguished without the ability to identify the orders within the sequences (or even the component sounds themselves).

It is suggested that we employ two quite different processes for distinguishing between permuted orders of sounds within extended sequences: 1) direct identification of components and their orders; and 2) holistic pattern recognition. Direct identification of components and their orders is limited by the time required for the verbal labeling (naming) of sounds, and requires at least 100 msec per item for speech sounds and at least 200 msec per item for nonrelated sounds. Sequences consisting of the same sounds in different orders can be discriminated through a holistic pattern recognition at item durations too brief to permit direct identification of order. Following holistic pattern recognition of familiar sequences, listeners may be able to recite by rote the names of components in their order of occurrence—however, this process should not be confused with direct identification of components and their order. As will be discussed in chapter 7, speech perception appears to be based on holistic pattern recognition.

6

Perceptual Restoration of Missing Sounds

The world is a noisy place, and sounds of importance are often accompanied by irrelevant noise. Hearing would lose much of its usefulness could we discern only whichever sound was at the highest level. However, there are mechanisms permitting us to attend to fainter sounds. In addition, we can, under certain circumstances, perceptually restore sounds which have been obliterated completely.

Mechanisms capable of separating fainter from louder sounds have been discussed in chapter 2. One is associated with localization, and reduces the threshold for a sound at one place when subject to interference by a sound at a different location. Another mechanism squelches or reduces the interference produced by reverberation through isolation of components reaching the listener directly from the source.

Nevertheless, signals of importance can still be completely masked. But when masking is intermittent so that snatches of the signal furnish information concerning the missing segments, perceptual synthesis may result in listeners hearing the missing sounds as clearly as those actually present. As we shall see, such perceptual synthesis is appropriate not only to the context provided by the unmasked fragments, but also to the masking potential of the extraneous sound: that is, restoration requires that the interfering sound have the intensity and spectral characteristics necessary to mask the sound which is restored.

TEMPORAL INDUCTION

The general term "auditory induction" has been proposed for processes leading to the restoration of obliterated signals (Warren & Bashford, 1976; Warren, Obusek, & Ackroff, 1972). There has been a discussion in chapter 2 of "contralateral induction" which can permit restoration of monaurally masked signals, and prevent mislocalization of a source at the side of the unmasked ear. The present chapter will deal with "temporal induction" which permits restoration of signals subject to intermittent masking on the basis of information provided by prior and subsequent portions of the signal.

Homophonic Continuity

Perhaps the simplest form of temporal induction is what has been called "homophonic" continuity (Warren, Obusek, & Ackroff, 1972). This effect was heard originally while the first author was listening through headphones to a recycled sequence of three successive intensity levels (60, 70, 80 dB) of a band of noise one octave wide centered at 2,000 Hz, with each intensity level lasting for 300 msec. When this sequence was repeated without pause, the 60 dB level appeared to be on all the time, continuing through the 70 and 80 dB sounds. All listeners, whether psychoacoustically sophisticated or naive, heard the softest sound continuing along with each of the louder sounds. However, introduction of silent gaps of 50 msec between successive intensity levels destroyed the apparent continuity, and each of the three sounds were heard as separate bursts.

Homophonic continuity does not require that the repeated sequence consist of three intensities: it was found that alternation of 300 msec bursts of noise at 70 and 80 dB produced apparent continuity of the fainter sound. The absolute intensity levels and extent of intensity difference between the two levels did not appear to be critical variables (Warren et al., 1972). Any band of noise or any tone alternating between two intensity levels seemed to produce illusory continuity of the lower intensity level. However, when the intensity difference between the two levels of the sound was less than 3 dB (e.g., 80 dB alternating with 82 dB), the sound presented at the higher level appeared to be the fainter of the two sounds. That is, the 80 dB sound was heard to be on continuously, with the pulsed addition of a fainter sound corresponding to the presentation of the 82 dB sound. Let us examine the implication of the sound at the higher level being heard as fainter under these conditions.

Were the 80 dB noise actually on continuously with the intermittent addition of another 80 dB noise, the resultant intensity when both were present would be 83 dB. Indeed, when 80 dB and 83 dB levels of the same noise were alternated with each level lasting 300 msec, listeners did interpret the stimulus as the periodic addition of a sound equal in intensity to the continuous one. It appears that, when subjects are presented with 80 dB alternating with 82 dB, the perceptually continuous component of 80 dB is subtracted from the 82 dB sound leaving a residue of less than 80 dB (actually, subtracting 80 dB from 82 dB leaves 77.7 dB).

Homophonic continuity can be considered as a cancellation of masking, the listener using part of a louder sound for construction of a fainter sound.

As we shall see, illusory continuity is not restricted to sounds differing only in intensity, since "heterophonic" continuity can occur in which the restored sound differs in spectral composition from the louder sound. Further, restoration of sounds is not limited to maintenance of continuity: sounds differing from the preceding and following sounds can be restored under appropriate conditions, as will be discussed below. However, homophonic continuity represents an especially simple type of restoration for which the louder and fainter sounds differ only in intensity.

Heterophonic Continuity

The illusory continuation of one sound when replaced by a different, louder sound has been discovered independently by several investigators. Miller and Licklider (1950) seemed to have been the first to report this type of auditory induction. They found that if a tone was alternated with a louder broad-band noise (each sound lasting 50 msec), the tone appeared to be on all the time. Similar observations were made when they used word lists rather than tones: the voice appeared to be on continuously. However, missing phonemes were not restored, and intelligibility of the lists of monosyllabic words was not better than when the words were interrupted by silent gaps. Miller and Licklider stated that this illusory continuity was much like seeing a landscape through a picket fence when "... the pickets interrupt the view at regular intervals, but the landscape is perceived as continuing behind the pickets."

Vicario (1960) discovered illusory continuity independently. He called the illusion the "acoustic tunnel effect," again in analogy to vision. In the visual tunnel effect, which had been described by Gestalt psychologists, an object moving behind another appears to continue to exist behind (or within) the blocking object until it emerges on the other side.

Thurlow (1957) also rediscovered illusory continuity. He used two alternating tones differing in both intensity and frequency, and reported that the fainter tone could be heard to continue through 60 msec bursts of the louder tone. Thurlow described the phenomenon as "an auditory figure-ground effect" using the static model of Gestalt psychology's visual figure-ground effect, in which the background is assumed by viewers to extend behind a superimposed figure. Thurlow's work led to a series of studies on illusory continuity spanning gaps ranging from under 10 msec through 100 msec when these interruptions were filled with a louder sound (Elfner, 1969, 1971; Elfner & Caskey, 1965; Elfner & Homick, 1966, 1967a, 1967b; Thurlow & Elfner, 1959; Thurlow & Marten, 1962). Thurlow and Erchul (1978), on the basis of these studies as well as additional work, indicated their belief in the validity of the suggestion first made by Thurlow and Elfner (1959) that illusory continuity was a consequence of facilitation by the louder sound of a continued firing of the neural units corresponding to the fainter sound, this facilitation possibly arising through an excitatory post-synaptic potential. It should be noted that this model does not require that the louder sound be capable of stimulating directly the units responding to the fainter sound.

Houtgast (1972) used conditions producing longer illusory continuity than earlier studies, and obtained results suggesting to him a rather different hypothesis than that proposed by Thurlow and his colleagues. Houtgast considered that there was a close relation between illusory continuity and masking, and he suggested the following rule: "When a tone and a stimulus S are alternated (alternation cycle about 4 Hz), the tone is perceived as being continuous when the transition from S to tone causes no (perceptible) increase of nervous activity in any frequency region." He called the intensity at which perception of the tone changed from continuous to discontinuous the "pulsation threshold," and went on to say, "The pulsation threshold, thus, is the highest level of the tone at which this condition still holds." With the aid of some assumptions, Houtgast (1972, 1973, 1974b, 1974c) employed this illusory continuity to investigate cochlear spectral analysis. The basic reasoning underlying Houtgast's investigations was that lateral suppression took place on the basilar membrane as suggested by Békésy (1959). It was considered that lateral suppression, which reduced the extent of neural responses at the edges of stimulated regions, could not be studied directly by masking experiments (as had been tried by other investigators), since both the masker and the probe would be subject to the same suppression process. However, Houtgast believed that nonsimultaneous stimulation as used in illusory continuity experiments permitted an indirect measurement of the magnitude of lateral suppression.

At the same time as the initial report of Houtgast (1972), experiments involving heterophonic continuity of somewhat longer duration (300 msec) were reported by Warren, Obusek, and Ackroff (1972). They concluded, as did Houtgast, that illusory continuity of the fainter of two alternating sounds required that the louder sound be a potential masker of the fainter. However, they were influenced by earlier work dealing with phonemic restoration. It had been reported that, when a phoneme or group of phonemes in a sentence was replaced by a louder extraneous sound capable of masking the portion of the sentence it replaced, listeners restored the missing phoneme(s) and could not distinguish between the actual and perceptually synthesized speech sounds (Warren, 1970b). Since restoration does not appear to be restricted to continuity of a steady-state sound, Warren, Obusek, and Ackroff (1972) suggested that temporal induction could occur when the conditions of the following rule were met: "If there is contextual evidence that a sound may be present at a given time, and if the peripheral units stimulated by a louder sound include those which would be stimulated by the anticipated fainter sound, then the fainter sound may be heard as present." This rule considers that with sufficient contextual support, any missing portion of an auditory pattern may be perceptually synthesized when it is replaced by a potential masker. This restoration can lead not only to apparent continuity of a steady sound, as in Houtgast's rule, but to phonemic restorations, continuity of tonal glides, completion of musical phrases, etc.

In order to study the quantitative relation between masking and perceptual restoration, a detailed experiment was undertaken by Warren and his colleagues involving illusory continuity of sinusoidal tones. The inducing sound in the study was always a 1,000 Hz tone at 80 dB SPL which alternated with a fainter tone having the frequencies shown in figure 6.1. Each tone was on for 300 msec and off for 300 msec, and the six subjects were instructed to adjust the intensity of the fainter tone to the highest level at which it seemed to be on continuously. Listening was through diotically wired matched headphones. The triangular data points in the figure show the highest level permitting temporal induction at each frequency, the level being expressed as Sensation Level (dB above the subject's threshold). It can be seen that virtually no temporal induction occurred until the frequency of the fainter tone was above 700 Hz, so that for these lower frequencies, as long as the tone was loud enough to be heard clearly, it was perceived to be pulsing.

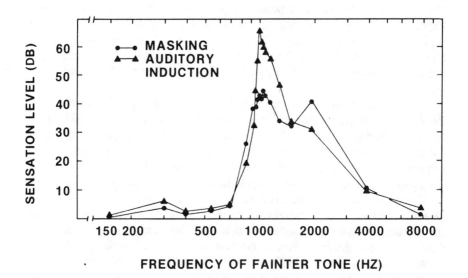

FREQUENCY OF FAINTER TONE (HZ)

Fig. 6.1. Temporal induction and masking for tones from 150 Hz through 8,000 Hz in the presence of a louder 1,000 Hz tone presented at 80 dB SPL.
Source: Adapted from R.M. Warren, C.J. Obusek, and J.M. Ackroff, "Auditory Induction: Perceptual Synthesis of Absent Sounds," *Science* 176 (1972): 1149-51. Copyright 1972 by the American Association for the Advancement of Science.

When the weaker tone was 1,000 Hz (the same frequency as the stronger tone), homophonic continuity took place. Most of the subjects chose a 3 dB difference in level between the 1,000 Hz tones as the upper limits of homophonic continuity since, as discussed earlier, the tone having the greater physical intensity appeared to be weaker than the continuous tone of the same frequency when the difference in intensity was less than 3 dB (the instructions specified an adjustment to the limit of illusory continuity of the *fainter* tone). While temporal induction increased sharply from 700 through 1,000 Hz, there was a relatively gradual decrease in temporal induction as frequencies increased above 1,000 Hz.

Simultaneous masking was measured using the same subjects. The 1,000 Hz tone was kept on continuously at 80 dB SPL, and the threshold was measured for detection of pulsed superimposed tones which were on for 300 msec and off for 300 msec. The data points shown by circles in figure 6.1 give the simultaneous masking thresholds in terms of Sensation Level (deciBels above the detection threshold) for the fainter sound when alternated with the louder one. The figure shows that the masking and temporal induction functions were quite similar up to 975 Hz. When the fainter stimulus was 1,000 Hz, maxima occurred for both the apparent continuity and the masking functions. At identical inducer and inducee frequencies, as indicated earlier, temporal induction became homophonic, and also the threshold for masking became a special kind of masking equivalent to a just noticeable difference in intensity. The functions for apparent continuity and masking were the same at 1,500 Hz and above, except for one frequency. There was a separation in the two functions at 2,000 Hz due to an increase in the masked threshold. This increase in masking one octave above the frequency of a tonal masker has been known for some time (Wegel and Lane, 1924), and was discussed in chapter 4. It can be seen in the figure that a change in slope also occurs in the temporal induction curve at 2,000 Hz, but the magnitude of this change is appreciably less than that of the masking curve.

Warren and his colleagues reported additional observations providing evidence indicating a close relation between temporal induction and masking. They used a 1/3-octave band noise centered on 1,000 Hz as the inducing sound, and found that the upper intensity limit for illusory continuity of tones was highest for the tonal frequency corresponding to the center frequency of the noise band. As with the tonal inducer shown in figure 6.1, the curve describing the intensity limits for temporal induction of the tone by the noise band was asymmetrical with steeper slopes at the low frequency end. A broad-band noise with a frequency notch (that is, a rejected frequency band) centered on 1,000 Hz also was used. In keeping with the hypothesized relation between masking and temporal induction, the upper intensity limit for apparent continuity of tones was lowest at the center frequency of this rejected noise band.

The Roll Effect as Tonal Restoration

Van Noorden (1975, 1977) discovered that, when faint 40 msec tone bursts were alternated with louder 40 msec tone bursts with short silent gaps separating the successive bursts, it was possible for listeners to hear the fainter tone burst not only when it actually was present, but also whenever the louder burst occurred. This "roll effect" resulted in an apparent doubling of the actual rate of the fainter bursts, and required intensity and spectral relations between fainter and louder tones resembling those leading to illusory continuity of the fainter of two alternating temporally contiguous tones. As van Noorden pointed out, it was as if the discrete restorations of the fainter tonal bursts leading to the roll effect required that the louder bursts could function as potential maskers.

Temporal Limits for Illusory Continuity

Studies of the illusory continuity of tones all have used interruption times of 300 msec or less, since tonal continuity cannot be maintained for longer periods. (See Verschuure, 1978, for a discussion of temporal limits for the continuity of tones.) However, an extremely long-lasting continuity was reported by Warren et al. (1972) for a 1/3-octave band of noise centered on 1,000 Hz when alternated with a louder 500 to 2,000 Hz band of pink noise of equal duration. All of their 15 subjects heard the fainter noise band continue for several seconds, 8 heard illusory continuity for at least 20 seconds, and 6 still were hearing the absent noise band continue 50 seconds after it was replaced by the broad-band noise.

Illusory Continuity of Stimuli Repeated at Tonal and Infratonal Frequencies

Illusory continuity of tones has been used to measure characteristics of spectral (place) analysis (see Fastl, 1975; Houtgast, 1972; Kronberg, Mellert, & Schreiner, 1974; Rodenburg & Maas, 1974; Verschuure, 1974, 1977, 1978). However, there is reason to believe that both spectral and temporal analyses contribute to the illusory continuity of periodic sounds.

A recent unpublished study by Warren, Wrightson, and Puretz was designed to determine if illusory continuity could be heard for periodic sounds repeated at infratonal frequencies. Since iteration can be detected only through neural temporal analysis at these frequencies, illusory continuity would involve temporal domain information. It was reasoned that, if illusory infrapitch continuity took place, then explanations for illusory continuity of tones based solely on place information might be incomplete. Iterated noise segments were chosen as stimuli, in keeping with the suggestion that randomly derived waveforms can serve as model periodic stimuli (see chapter 3). Both infratonal and tonal frequencies were used, with the stimuli covering the range from 10 through 2,000 Hz. The periodic sounds had adjustable intensities, and were alternated with on-line noise at a fixed level of 80 dB. Each sound was on for 300 msec and off for 300 msec, and the four subjects listened to the stimuli delivered diotically through matched headphones. All sounds were low-pass filtered at 8,000 Hz and, for iterated noise segments of 50 Hz and above, both the periodic stimulus and the on-line noise were high-pass filtered at the fundamental frequency of the recycled noise. The subjects were instructed to adjust the fainter periodic sound to the highest level at which the periodicity could be heard as continuous. Illusory continuity of iterance was heard by all subjects for all repetition frequencies. Continuity could be heard at higher sensation levels in the infratonal range (iterance subserved solely by neural temporal mechanisms) than in the tonal range, with the intensity limit for temporal induction decreasing regularly with increasing frequency. It would appear that temporal mechanisms are capable of sustaining an illusory persistance of iterance, and that explanations offered for tonal continuity solely in terms of spectral mechanisms may be inadequate.

Incomplete Continuity or Illusory Lengthening

The upper duration limit for illusory continuity, or pulsation threshold, appears as a fairly sharp break, enabling reproducible measures to be made of this transition (Fastl, 1975; Schreiner, Gottlob, & Mellert, 1977; Verschuure, Rodenburg, & Maas, 1974). However, a recent study by Wrightson and Warren (1981) indicated that measurable illusory lengthening can occur when the fainter sound does not appear to be continuous. In this study, subjects judged apparent offset times and onset times of a 70 dB sinusoidal tone having a duration of one second which was alternated with a narrow band of 80 dB noise having a center frequency of 1,000 Hz and a duration of 500 msec. Tone bursts and noise bursts were temporally contiguous, with 5 msec switching rise/fall times (i.e., upon switching, the intensities of the tone and noise each changed at a rate of 60 dB per 5 msec). For tonal frequencies corresponding to those within the noiseband, apparent tonal offset was late by an average of 112 msec and apparent tonal onset early by an average of 101 msec. For all frequencies of the tone outside the noiseband's range, both onset and offset judgments were much more accurate. It should be noted that the illusory lengthening occurs in directions opposite to those corresponding to backward masking and forward masking. Backward masking should cause the offset to appear early, and forward masking should cause the onset to appear late, thus shortening rather than lengthening the apparent duration of the tone. Warren, Obusek, and Ackroff (1972) had found that brief (50 msec)

silent periods between alternating fainter and louder sounds prevented temporal induction, and Wrightson and Warren observed that 50 msec of silence
between tone and noise also prevented errors in judgments corresponding to
late offset and early onset.

Continuity can be considered as the limit of temporal expansion. It
seems that, as spectral and intensity requirements for illusory continuity are
approached, the apparent offset of the fainter sound occurs later and its
apparent onset occurs earlier until the perception of interruption is lost
abruptly when the gap is bridged completely.

Illusory Pattern Completion: Restoration of Frequency Glides

Dannenbring (1976) studied the illusory continuity of tonal glides interrupted
by noise. An example of the stimulus used is shown in figure 6.2. The
difference in frequency between the upper and lower limits of the glide range
was varied from 100 through 1,000 Hz (the center frequency of the glide range
always was 1,000 Hz), and the duration of the glide from frequency peak to
trough was varied from 250 through 2,000 msec. The duration of white noise
bursts centered at the middle of each glide was adjusted by the subjects to the
maximum duration permitting the glide to appear continuous. The stimuli
were presented diotically, with the noise burst at 90dB and the tonal glide at
75 dB. Illusory continuity of somewhat longer duration was found as ΔF (the
range of the frequency glide) increased. For the longest duration glide (two
seconds from peak to trough), the tonal glide was heard to continue smoothly
through noise durations between 400 and 500 msec (mean of adjustments for
the 20 subjects) for each value of ΔF.

Glides require completion of a pattern which differs at the beginning and
end of the signal interruption. While perceptual synthesis of contextually
appropriate sounds differing from those present at the time of interruption
had been reported for phonemic restorations, Dannenbring's study demonstrates that such perceptual syntheses can occur with nonverbal stimuli as
well. Restorations of frequency glides and of missing phonemes are not in
keeping with the model of Thurlow and his colleagues (Thurlow & Elfner,
1959; Thurlow & Erchul, 1978) which considers perceptual restoration in
terms of a mechanism permitting continuity of ongoing neural activity.
Another difficulty for this theory is the observation by Wrightson and Warren
(1981) who, as described above, reported that, under conditions leading to a
partial continuation of a tonal signal alternated with noise, the tone seemed to
start about 100 msec before its actual beginning. A theory based on persistence of neural activity cannot explain readily the premature apparent onset of
the tone.

One further difficulty for the neural persistence theory of illusory continuity applied to single sounds was described by Bregman and Dannenbring (1977). They studied the effects of amplitude ramps which either increased or decreased the intensity of a fainter tone of fixed frequency for brief periods (50 msec or less) before the introduction of a louder broad-band noise burst, and found that the increasing intensity ramp decreased apparent continuity (although to a lesser extent than the decreasing ramp). They reasoned that a simple neural persistence model would predict that an increasing intensity

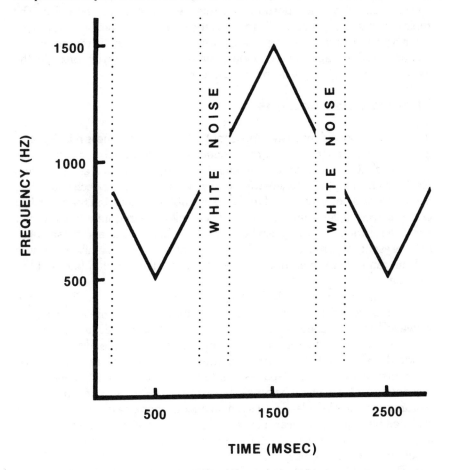

Fig. 6.2. Example of conditions used to study illusory continuity (temporal induction) of tonal glides interrupted by louder broad-band noise.
Source: Modified from G.L. Dannenbring, "Perceived Auditory Continuity with Alternately Rising and Falling Frequency Transitions," *Canadian Journal of Psychology* 30 (1976): 99-114.

ramp should facilitate tonal continuity across the noise-filled interruption, and concluded that their experimental results provided evidence against such a model.

TEMPORAL INDUCTION OF SPEECH

There are three classes of studies dealing with the temporal induction of speech occurring when portions are replaced (or masked) by noise. The topics dealt with in these studies are: (1) the nature of phonemic restorations when a portion of speech is replaced by a single noise burst; (2) the increase in "naturalness" or apparent continuity with multiple interruptions; (3) the increase in intelligibility with multiple interruptions.

Phonemic Restorations

It has been reported that listeners cannot tell that a phoneme is missing after it has been excised from a recorded sentence and replaced by an extraneous sound such as a cough or a noise burst (Warren, 1970b; Warren & Warren, 1970). Even when the listeners were told in advance that a speech sound had been removed completely and replaced by another sound and the recording was replayed several times, the sentence still appeared intact; it was not possible for them to distinguish between the absent sound and those physically present (Warren & Obusek, 1971). However, when a silent gap was present rather than an extraneous sound, the missing speech sound could be identified.

It might be thought that listeners could identify the position of the extraneous sound in the sentence, and thus locate the missing segment. However, the extraneous sound could not be localized accurately: when subjects attempted to report its position, errors corresponding to a few hundred milliseconds were made. Similar observations were reported for phonemic restorations in Japanese sentences by Sasaki (1980). Sasaki also reasoned that there might be a melodic restoration effect similar to phonemic restorations. He did indeed find such an effect: when one or two notes were replaced by noise in familiar melodies played at a moderate rate on a piano, listeners heard the missing note(s), and mislocalized the noise burst when required to report its location.

The inability to locate extraneous sounds in sentences and melodies is consistent with reports of a general inability to detect order directly in other sequences with equivalent item durations (see chapter 5). Although the phonemes forming sentences and the notes forming musical passages may occur too rapidly to permit direct naming of order, verbal and melodic groupings can be recognized holistically. Following recognition of the overall pattern, the identity and order of components forming these sequences can be inferred. This indirect mechanism for naming orders at rates too rapid for direct identification of sounds and their orders is not available for locating the position of extraneous sounds within familiar sequences.

Both phonemic and melodic restorations can be considered as highly specialized forms of temporal induction, with the nature of the induced sound determined by the special rules governing these sequences. In keeping with the general rule found to govern temporal induction, there is evidence that restoration of a phoneme can be enhanced when the extraneous sound in a sentence is capable of masking the restored speech sound (Layton, 1975; Samuel, 1981a). Restoration of single phonemes in sentences has been used to study mechanisms for perceptual organization of speech, and will be discussed further in chapter 7.

Apparent Continuity of Speech Produced by Insertion of Noise into Gaps

Miller and Licklider (1950) reported that, when recordings of PB ("phonetically balanced") lists of monosyllabic words were interrupted regularly by silent gaps at rates from 10 to 15 times a second (50 percent duty cycle, so that on-time and off-time were equal), the silent intervals caused the voice to sound rough and harsh, and intelligibility dropped. When the silent gaps were filled with a broad-band noise which was louder than the speech, Miller and Licklider found that the speech sounded more "natural" (their "picket fence effect") but intelligibility was no better than it was with silence. Bashford and Warren (1979) extended this study of the effects of filling silent gaps with noise, using three types of recorded verbal stimuli: (1) PB word lists of the type employed by Miller and Licklider; (2) an article from a popular news magazine read backwards (the individual words were pronounced normally, but they were read in reverse order with an attempt to preserve normal phrasing contours); (3) the same magazine article read in a normal fashion. The rate at which syllables occurred was matched for all three stimuli, which were presented at peak intensity levels of 70 dB. Twenty listeners adjusted the interruption rate of the verbal stimuli (50 percent duty cycle, rise/fall time of 10 msec) to the minimum value at which they could perceive that portions of the signal were missing. Under one condition the gaps were unfilled, and under the other condition the gaps were filled with broad-band pink noise at 80 dB. (Pink noise has equal power per octave, and resembles the long-term average of the spectral distribution of power in speech.) Table 6.1 lists the deletion detection thresholds obtained in this study.

Table 6.1. Deletion detection thresholds (msec) for a group of 20 subjects.

	Normal Discourse	Discourse Read Backwards	PB Words
Noise	304.4	147.7	161.5
Silence	52.0	50.0	61.5

Source: From J.A. Bashford, Jr., and R.M. Warren, "Perceptual Synthesis of Deleted Phonemes," in *Speech Communication Papers,* edited by J.J. Wolf and D.H. Klatt (New York: Acoustical Society of America, 1979), pp. 423-26.

When speech was interrupted by silent gaps having durations less than the deletion detection threshold, it sounded rough or "bubbly," but perceptually discrete gaps were not heard. When each type of verbal stimulus was interrupted by noise for durations less than the deletion detection threshold, listeners reported that the signals sounded like fully continuous speech, with the noise bursts appearing to be superimposed (in keeping with the observations of Miller and Licklider with word lists). It can be seen that detection thresholds for silent gaps were similar for all three types of verbal signals. However, filling gaps with noise caused a considerable increase in the threshold value for recognition of discontinuities in the speech for all conditions, with the greatest increase occurring for normal discourse. These results suggest that temporal induction of continuity occurs with verbal as with other auditory stimuli, and that the extent of this verbal temporal induction is enhanced by the use of normal speech.

If the enhanced continuity of verbal stimuli is indeed based upon temporal induction, it should exhibit the spectral dependency demonstrated for temporal induction with nonverbal stimuli (i.e., the noise capable of inducing continuity should be capable of masking the speech were this signal really continuous). Bashford and Warren filtered the recording of normal speech described above to produce a 1/3-octave band centered on 1,500 Hz. This filtered speech was presented at peak levels of 70 dB and alternated with 1/3-octave bands of noise at 80 dB, having the center frequencies shown in figure 6.3. (Filter slopes were 48 dB per octave for speech and for noise.) The deletion detection thresholds were determined using the procedure described above for broad-band speech alternated with broad-band noise. The results demonstrate that the greatest enhancement of continuity occurred with spectral congruence of noise and speech, in keeping with temporal induction studies using other sounds.

Increase in Intelligibility of Speech Produced by Insertion of Noise into Gaps: Multiple Phonemic Restorations

As mentioned earlier, Miller and Licklider (1950) found that, although their recorded word lists sounded more natural when interruptions were filled with louder noise rather than being silent, no increase in intelligibility occurred with the introduction of noise. However, later investigators, who used meaningful discourse rather than word lists, did find that an increase in intelligibility was produced by insertion of noise into gaps in speech. Cherry and Wiley (1967) appear to be the first to report such an increase in intelligibility. They passed only the strongly voiced components of speech, and reported that the resultant stacatto sequence of high energy voiced speech sounds had an "extremely low intelligibility." But when noise of appropriate intensity was

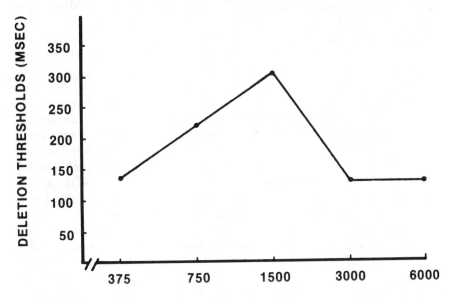

CENTER FREQUENCY OF INTERRUPTING
NOISE BAND (HZ)

Fig. 6.3. Deletion detection thresholds for filtered speech (narrow-band, center frequency 1,500 Hz) interrupted by louder narrow-band noise with various center frequencies.

Source: From J.A. Bashford, Jr., and R.M. Warren, "Perceptual Synthesis of Deleted Phonemes," in *Speech Communication Papers,* edited by J.J. Wolf and D.H. Klatt (New York: Acoustical Society of America, 1979), pp. 423-26.

added to the silent gaps, intelligibility increased considerably (from 20 percent to 70 percent). These basic findings were confirmed by Holloway (1970). Wiley (1968) reversed the procedure employed by Cherry and Wiley and by Holloway, and removed the strongly voiced components of running speech, leaving only the low energy speech sounds, and found again that intelligibility was increased when noise was added to the silent gaps. Wiley also deleted portions of the speech at regular intervals, and reported that once more intelligibility was increased by the addition of noise to gaps. Powers and Wilcox (1977) were not aware of Wiley's unpublished dissertation, and discovered independently that addition of noise to silent gaps in regularly interrupted speech increased intelligibility.

The enhancement of intelligibility produced by filling silent gaps of interrupted speech with noise has given rise to a number of hypotheses concerning its basis. Cherry and Wiley (1967) suggested that noise prevents some disruptive effect of silence upon a natural rhythm which is needed for comprehension. Powers and Wilcox (1977) concluded that their results were consistent with the rhythm hypothesis of Cherry and Wiley. In addition, they mentioned as another possible basis for enhanced intelligibility a suggestion made by Huggins (1964) that noise might serve to mask misleading transitions to silence which are known to produce illusory consonants. However, this latter suggestion is weakened by the observation that illusory consonants are produced also by the introduction of silent gaps in isolated monosyllables (Öhman, 1966), yet no improvement in intelligibility occurs when noise is inserted into such gaps if the words do not form connected speech (Dirks & Bower, 1970; Miller & Licklider, 1950). Warren and Obusek (1971) hypothesized that multiple phonemic restorations were produced by introduction of noise into gaps generated by deleting portions of connected speech, with the mechanisms for restoring phonemes utilizing semantic and syntactic context concerning the identity of the missing fragments. Bashford and Warren (1979) attempted to determine if multiple phonemic restorations were indeed involved by testing for the dependence of intelligibility enhancement on the spectral characteristics of the noise. If phonemic restorations can be considered as a special linguistic form of temporal induction, then intelligibility should be enhanced by a spectral matching of speech and noise.

Bashford and Warren instructed a group of 20 listeners to repeat standardized lists of sentences developed at the Central Institute for the Deaf (Silverman & Hirsh, 1955) which were presented in filtered form (1/3-octave filter with slopes of 48 dB per octave, center frequency of 1,500 Hz) and interrupted periodically at two interruptions per second (250 msec on/off times with 10 msec rise/fall time). The gaps in the sentence were filled with one of five 1/3-octave bands of noise (48 dB per octave slopes) with center frequencies as shown in figure 6.3. The speech was presented at a peak level of 70 dB with noise bands at 80 dB, and listening was through diotically wired

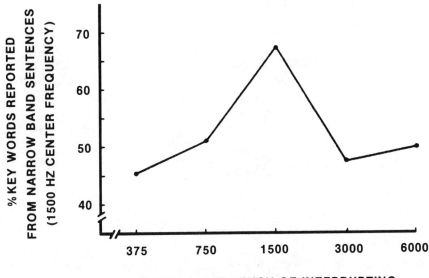

Fig. 6.4. Intelligibility scores for filtered sentences (narrow-band, center frequency 1,500 Hz) interrupted by louder narrow-band noise with various center frequencies.
Source: From J.A. Bashford, Jr., and R.M. Warren, "Perceptual Synthesis of Deleted Phonemes," in *Speech Communication Papers*, edited by J.J. Wolf and D.H. Klatt (New York: Acoustical Society of America, 1979): 423-26.

headphones. The results of the intelligibility test are shown in figure 6.4. It can be seen that intelligibility was greatest when the noise band and speech band were spectrally matched as would be expected from temporal induction theory.

MASKING AND UNMASKING

While masking seems to be an apt term for describing the perceptual obliteration of one signal by another, considering temporal induction as the unmasking of a signal can be misleading. Unmasking suggests drawing aside a curtain of noise to reveal the intact signal. But the truly masked signal is no more, and any restoration must be considered a recreation or perceptual synthesis of the contextually appropriate sound.

Illusory continuity of a single sound interrupted by noise is an especially simple form of perceptual synthesis, and phonemic restorations a highly skilled and complex type of synthesis drawing upon linguistic rules. The nature of these rules is discussed in the following chapter on speech.

7

Speech

Earlier chapters dealing with nonlinguistic auditory perception treated humans as receivers and processors of acoustic information. But when dealing with speech perception, it is necessary also to consider humans as generators of acoustic signals. The two topics of speech production and speech perception are closely linked, as we shall see.

We shall deal first with the generation of speech sounds and the nature of the acoustic signals. The topic of speech perception will then be described in relation to general principles, which are applicable to nonspeech sounds as well as to speech. Finally, the topic of special perceptual strategies employed for perception of speech will be explored.

SPEECH PRODUCTION

The structures used for producing speech have evolved from organs that served other functions in our prelinguistic ancestors and still perform nonlinguistic functions in humans.

It is convenient to divide the system for production of speech into three regions (see Fig. 7.1). The subglottal system delivers air under pressure to the larynx (located behind the Adam's apple) which contains a pair of vocal folds (also called vocal cords). The opening between the vocal folds is called the glottis, and the rapid opening and closing of the glottal slit interrupts the air flow, resulting in a buzz-like sound. The buzz is then spectrally shaped to form speech sounds or phonemes by the supralaryngeal vocal tract having the larynx at one end and the lips and the nostrils at the other. In addition to modifying the laryngeal buzz, the vocal tract also is used to produce noises and plosive sounds with phonetic significance.

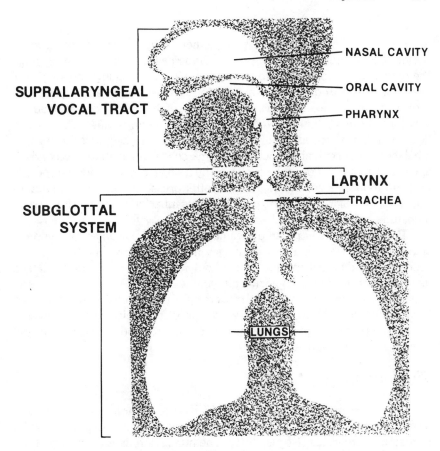

Fig. 7.1. Anatomical structures involved in speech production. The subglottal system delivers air under pressure to the larynx. The vocal folds in the larynx are capable of generating broad-band sounds. The supraglottal system can spectrally shape the sound produced in the larynx by altering dimensions along the vocal tract, and by opening or closing access to the nasal passages. The supraglottal system is also capable of adding some hisses and pops of its own.

The Subglottal System

The glottis remains open during normal breathing without phonation. Inhalation is accomplished through expansion of the chest cavity, largely through contraction of the diaphragm and the external intercostal muscles. Exhalation is accomplished mainly through elastic recoil when the contraction of the muscles used for inhalation ceases. However, during more active breathing, including that accompanying speaking, the passive compression of air in the lungs following active inhalation is supplemented by contraction of the internal intercostal and abdominal muscles. The air passes from the lungs through the windpipe or trachea up to the larynx. During speaking, the subglottal pressure is usually equivalent to about 5 to 10 cm of water (that is, equal to the force per unit area exerted by a water column of this height), although during very loud shouting it can rise to the equivalent of 60 cm of water. The average flow rates during speech are roughly 150 to 200 cm³/sec, and the average inhalation for speech about 500 to 800 cm³, so that up to about 5 seconds of speech or about 15 words are produced by a single breath in normal speech. Delicate muscular control of the subglottal pressure and flow rate appropriate to particular articulatory gestures is essential for generating the normal amplitude patterns of speech.

Production of all English phonemes is powered by subglottal compression of air. However, there are languages in which some of the phonemes are produced by different means. A rapid downward movement of the closed glottis is used to create implosive phonemes in some American Indian and African languages, and an upward movement of the closed glottis can be used to produce "ejective" pops and hisses with phonetic significance. Movements of the tongue to suck air into the mouth are used to produce clicks in several languages of southern Africa.

The Larynx

The larynx is homologous with a valve which protects the lungs of the lungfish from flooding, and is used generally for phonation or sound production by terrestrial vertebrates (Negus, 1949). The human larynx is at the top of the trachea and houses vocal folds consisting of two strips of ligaments and muscles attached to a firm cartilagenous support. During swallowing, the epiglottis moves down to seal off the larynx while solid and liquid material is moved into the esophagus. During normal breathing without phonation, the glottal opening between the vocal folds remains in a half-open position, although it can be opened more fully during rapid intake of breath. During voicing or phonation, the vocal folds open and close rhythmically to produce puffs of air. These puffs correspond to a buzz-like periodic sound which furnishes the raw acoustic substrate from which vowels and voiced consonants are shaped. The harmonic components of the buzz decrease in amplitude with increasing frequency, so that there is roughly equal power per octave. During whispering, the vocal folds are kept in a nearly closed position, creating turbulence and a corresponding hiss-like sound, which is shaped by the supraglottal region as is the glottal buzz of voiced sounds. Whispered speech also can be produced by other constrictions leading to hisses at positions near the laryngeal end of the vocal tract.

The opening and closing of the vocal folds are not synchronous with muscle twitches as once thought by some investigators but, rather, follow from the effects of rapid air flow through the glottis. During normal phonation, prevoicing changes in muscle tension cause the vocal folds to move close together. The relatively high velocity of air past the constriction produced by the vocal folds causes a drop in air pressure at their edges, and Bernoulli's principle (that is, an increase in a fluid's velocity causes a decrease in its pressure) causes the vocal folds to be drawn together, and to close. The closure results in a build-up of subglottal pressure, forcing the vocal folds open, releasing a puff of air which causes the cycle to repeat for as long as phonation is maintained.

Much information about the operation of the vocal folds has been obtained by direct observation. By placing a mirror at the appropriate angle at the back of the throat, it is possible both to illuminate and to view glottal configurations (see Fig. 7.2). Since movements are rapid during phonation, a high-speed motion picture camera is very useful for studying the cycle of opening and closing during voicing. Some pictures of a single period of vocal fold vibration are shown in figure 7.2. The entire vibratory period shown in the figure occupied 1/140 sec.

The rate at which the glottis opens and closes is the voice's fundamental frequency, and determines the pitch. The rate of glottal vibration is under the control of several sets of muscles which can raise the pitch by increasing the length and hence the tension of the vocal folds. The intensity of the voice can be controlled by changing both the subglottal pressure and the portion of the glottal period during which the vocal cords are open. Decreasing the portion of the cycle during which the vocal folds are open results in a louder sound as well as a change in quality associated with a greater vocal effort.

The fundamental frequency of the voice is about 120 Hz for an adult male and about 250 Hz for an adult female. Children may have fundamental frequencies as high as 400 Hz. The low frequency in adult males is associated with thickening and lengthening of the vocal folds resulting from hormonal changes occurring at puberty. The range of frequencies employed in speech by male and female adults is usually a little more than one octave, with a modal frequency about 1/3-octave above the lower limit of this range.

The trained voice of a singer exhibits exceptionally fine control of pitch, loudness, and quality of phonation. There are three sets of intrinsic laryngeal muscles which are "synergistic" in terms of fundamental frequency and intensity (Hirano, Ohala, & Vennard, 1969): while untrained people often change intensity when they change their fundamental frequency, trained singers can alter intensity and frequency independently. Singers deliberately introduce an instability or periodic fluctuation in pitch called the vibrato, which is centered upon the frequency corresponding to the sung note. (The

START

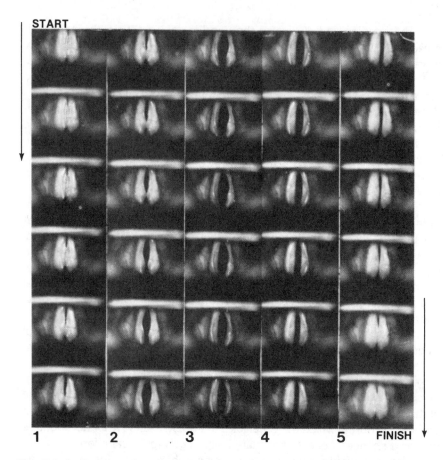

1   2   3   4   5   FINISH

Fig. 7.2. A single cycle of vocal-fold vibration taken with a high-speed film
exposed at 4,000 frames per second.
Source: From W.R. Zemlin, *Speech and Hearing Science: Anatomy and
Physiology* (2nd Ed.), © 1981, p. 151. Reproduced by permission of
Prentice-Hall, Inc., Englewood Cliffs, N.J.

frequency of this fluctuation is about six or seven per second, and the
frequency excursion as large as one semitone.) The extraction of a single
pitch by a listener from this ever-changing frequency involves not a moment-
by-moment evaluation but, rather, an averaging over time. The vibrato is a
fairly recent development in our culture: even in the nineteenth century, the
ability to sing notes with a fixed pitch was a difficult and admired ability of
trained singers. Operatic singers also occasionally use tremolo which consists of an irregular amplitude modulation superimposed upon the frequency
modulation of the vibrato.

Singers usually are capable of producing a range of pitches well beyond that used in speech. In order to cover this range, they employ a number of different production modes, each corresponding to a different "register." Thus, the falsetto register (used by male singers in reaching their highest notes) involves a tensing of the vocal folds so that only a portion of the edges vibrate; the "laryngeal whistle" register (used by female singers in reaching their highest notes) does not involve vibration of the vocal folds but, instead, a whistle is produced by air passing through a small opening in the otherwise closed vocal folds. One of the goals of voice training is to permit transitions between different registers to be made smoothly and, ideally, without the listener being able to detect a discontinuity in the passage from one to another. A trained soprano may be able to use fundamental frequencies covering the range from 130 through 2,000 Hz by employing the so-called "chest register" below 300 Hz, the "head voice" from about 300 to 1,000 Hz, the "little register" from about 1,000 to 1,500 Hz, and the "whistle register" above 1,500 Hz. (For a discussion of the various registers and theories concerning their production see Deinse, 1981.)

While people are quite unaware of the mechanisms employed for changing pitch in speaking, it might be thought that singers would have insight into their methods for pitch change, since so much time and effort is devoted to studying this topic. Yet, there is available only a rather vague and ambiguous vocabulary describing the registers and qualities of the singing voice. The location of the muscles employed and their delicate control through acoustic, tactile, and proprioceptive (muscular) feedback is accomplished with little or no direct knowledge on the part of the performer, providing an example of what Polanyi (1958, 1968) has called "tacit knowledge." However, the ability to describe the muscular activity employed in vocal production increases as we move down the airstream from larynx to lips, as will be discussed later when we deal with the perceptual status of the phoneme.

The Vocal Tract and Articulation of Speech Sounds

The buzz produced by the larynx becomes speech only after being modified by its passage through the vocal tract. During this trip, phonemes are formed by the spectral shaping of the laryngeal buzz, and by obstructing the airflow. A highly simplified model of the vocal tract considers it to be a tube, like an organ pipe, which is open at one end. In a male, the length of this tube is about 17.5 cm. As an initial simplifying approximation, this tube can be considered to have a uniform cross-section. The lowest resonant frequency of such a tube has a wavelength four times the tube length, corresponding to about 500 Hz for a male. Those spectral components of the broad-band laryngeal source having frequencies of about 500 Hz are increased in intensity by this resonance to produce the first formant band. Additional resonances occur in the tube at odd-numbered integral multiples of the first formant, so that the second formant is at 1,500 Hz, and the third formant at 2,500 Hz. The vocal tracts of women are somewhat shorter, and the wavelengths associated with their corresponding formants are on the average about 80 to 85 percent of the male's. Formants are associated with standing waves (which correspond to fixed regions of high and low pressure), with all formants having one pressure maximum at the glottis and one pressure minimum at the lips. The first formant has only this one maximum and minimum, the second formant one additional maximum and minimum, and the third formant two additional maxima and minima, each spaced regularly along the uniform tube in this simplified model of the vocal tract.

However, vocal tracts are not uniform tubes. Not only can the tube be lengthened and shortened by movements of portions of the tract, but more importantly, cavities and constrictions can be created at the back of the throat and within the mouth. A decrease in cross-sectional area at a region of a formant's pressure amplitude minimum lowers the formant's frequency, while an increase in area at this region raises its frequency. Corresponding cross-sectional changes at places of pressure maxima have the opposite effect in changing the formant's frequency.

Vowels differ in the frequencies and relative intensities of their formants. Figure 7.3 shows the position of the vocal organs in producing extended statements of vowels. The procedure of preceding the vowel by /h/ and following it by /d/ minimizes the influence of adjacent phonemes, and produces vowels much like those produced in isolation. Table 7.1 gives the formant frequencies for the vowels shown in figure 7.3 as measured by Peterson and Barney (1952) for men, women, and children. The words used in speaking the vowels are given above their phonetic symbols. The single vowels shown are sometimes called monophthongs to distinguish them from diphthongs consisting of a pair such as /iu/occurring in the word "few."

Several cycles of a periodic sound such as a vowel are necessary to establish the fundamental and the line spectrum (see Fig. 1.1), and so it might be thought that a vowel could not be identified from a single glottal pulse. However, there have been reports that single glottal pulses, and even segments of pulses, can be used to identify vowels with accuracy not much below that found for extended statements (Gray, 1942; Moore & Mundie, 1971). Vowel recognition from a single pulse probably is based upon the distribution of spectral power in bands corresponding to the formants of extended vowel statements. Observations in my laboratory have indicated that conditions resembling those producing temporal induction (see chapter 6) can enhance the vowel-like characteristics of a single glottal pulse and facilitate its recognition. The procedure works well when the glottal pulse is preceded and followed by 1-second bursts of pink noise (that is, noise with equal power per octave) separated from the glottal pulse by no more than 5 msec of silence,

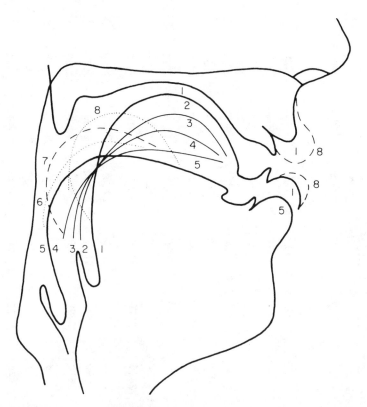

Fig. 7.3. Tongue positions for vowels in the words: (1) *heed,* (2) *hid,* (3) *head,* (4) *had,* (5) *hod,* (6) *hawed,* (7) *hood,* (8) *who'd.*
Source: From P.F. MacNeilage and P.Ladefoged, "The Production of Speech and Language," in E.C. Carterette and M. P. Friedman, *Handbook of Perception.* Vol. 7, *Language and Speech* (New York: Academic Press, 1976), pp. 75-120.

and presented at a level about 10 dB above that corresponding to the extended statement of the vowel from which the single pulse was excised.

Table 7.2 lists the English consonants by place and manner of articulation. All consonants involve some type of obstruction of the vocal tract. When accompanied by glottal vibration, they are voiced, otherwise they are unvoiced. Places of articulation are the lips (labial), teeth (dental), gums (alveolar), hard palate (palatal), soft palate (velar), and vocal folds or glottis (glottal). Stop consonants involve complete closure of the vocal tract. When the closure is followed by an audible release of air it is sometimes called a stop-plosive or, simply, plosive. Incomplete closure results in a fricative. When a stop is followed by a fricative, an affricative is produced (such as /t ʃ/ in "choice" and /d ʒ/ in "judge"). The glides (/r/, /w/, /j/, and /l/) are

Table 7.1 Averages of fundamental and formant frequencies and formant amplitudes of vowels by 33 men, 28 women, and 15 children.

		heed	hid	head	had	hod	hawed	hood	who'd
		i	I	ε	æ	ɑ	ɔ	ʊ	u
Fundamental frequencies (Hz)	M	136	135	130	127	124	129	137	141
	W	235	232	223	210	212	216	232	231
	Ch	272	269	260	251	256	263	276	274
Formant frequencies (Hz) F_1	M	270	390	530	660	730	570	440	300
	W	310	430	610	860	850	590	470	370
	Ch	370	530	690	1010	1030	680	560	430
F_2	M	2290	1990	1840	1720	1090	840	1020	870
	W	2790	2480	2330	2050	1220	920	1160	950
	Ch	3200	2730	2610	2320	1370	1060	1410	1170
F_3	M	3010	2550	2480	2410	2440	2410	2240	2240
	W	3310	3070	2990	2850	2810	2710	2680	2670
	Ch	3730	3600	3570	3320	3170	3180	3310	3260
Formant amplitudes (dB)	L_1	-4	-3	-2	-1	-1	0	-1	-3
	L_2	-24	-23	-17	-12	-5	-7	-12	-19
	L_3	-28	-27	-24	-22	-28	-34	-34	-43

Source: From G. E. Peterson and H. L. Barney, "Control Methods Used in a Study of the Vowels," *Journal of the Acoustical Society of America* 24 (1952): 115-84.

Table 7.2 Classification of English Consonants by Place and Manner of Articulation.

Place of Articulation	Stops Voiceless	Stops Voiced	Fricatives Voiceless	Fricatives Voiced	Nasals Voiceless	Nasals Voiced	Glides and Laterals Voiceless	Glides and Laterals Voiced
Labial	[p] (pin)	[b] (bin)				[m] (sum)	[hw] (what)	[w] (will)
Labiodental			[f] (fine)	[v] (vine)				
Dental			[θ] (thigh)	[ð] (thy)				
Alveolar	[t] (tin)	[d] (din)	[s] (sip)	[z] (zip)		[n] (sun)		[l] (less)
Palatal	[tʃ] (char)	[dʒ] (jar)	[ʃ] (ship)	[ʒ] (azure)				[j] (yes), [r] (rim)
Velar	[k] (kilt)	[g] (gilt)				[ŋ] (sung)		
Glottal			[h] (hill)					

Source: Adapted from W.R. Zemlin, *Speech and Hearing Science: Anatomy and Physiology* (2nd Ed.), © 1981, p. 359. Reproduced by permission of Prentice-Hall, Inc., Englewood Cliffs, N.J.

produced by rapid articulatory movements, and have characteristics in some ways intermediate between those of consonants and vowels. The nasal consonants are generated by blocking the passage of air through the mouth at the places characteristic of the consonant (see Table 7.2), with release of the air occurring through the nasal passages.

VISUAL REPRESENTATION OF SPEECH SOUNDS

The most direct way of representing the acoustic nature of speech is through its waveform. The waveform describes pressure changes over time. By construction of devices that record these changes in some mechanical or electrical fashion, we can use this record to recreate a more or less perfect copy of the original sound. Figure 7.4 shows the waveform corresponding to the word "poor."

While visual representations of waveforms have been used to characterize the speech stimulus, they have fallen out of favor in recent years. One reason is that the waveforms do not reveal the component harmonics or formants in any recognizable fashion. Waveforms of complex sounds do not correspond to the pattern of stimulation at any receptor site, since stimulation takes place only after a preliminary spectral analysis along the basilar membrane. It is possible to give an approximate description of the pattern of acoustic stimulation at individual receptor sites using multiple oscillograms corresponding to the output of a bank of filters, each filter having band-pass characteristics of a different critical band. Such tracings have some use in studying the perception of periodic sounds, as was discussed in chapter 3 and illustrated in figures 3.9, 3.11, 3.13, and 3.18. However, such a description of speech would be quite cumbersome, and would represent only a rough approximation of local stimulus patterns. A much more convenient description is furnished by sound spectrograms.

The sound spectrograph was developed at Bell Telephone Laboratories during the early 1940s. The device consists of a set of filters that are used successively to scan repetitions of a recorded speech sample (see Fig. 7.5). A sound spectrogram shows three variables: time is shown along the horizontal axis, frequency along the vertical axis, and intensity is shown by the darkness of the tracing. Figure 7.6 (a) shows a spectrogram of the phrase "to catch pink salmon." The formants of vowels are seen as dark horizontal bars. The silences of the stop consonants are shown as the vertical blank areas, and the fricative consonants correspond to the dark regions lacking discrete bars.

A group of workers at Haskins Laboratory developed a "pattern play-back" which can optically scan a sound spectrogram and recreate the original sounds. Using this device, it is possible to hand-paint patterns on a transparent base, and to play back the corresponding acoustic pattern to produce

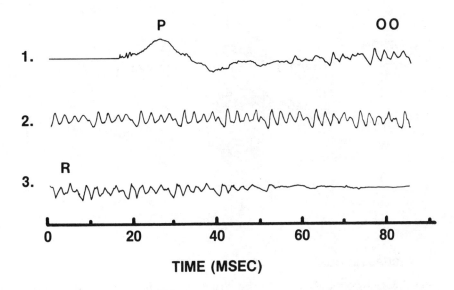

Fig. 7.4. Waveform of the word "poor." Three successive 85 msec segments are shown.
Source: From *Speech and Hearing in Communication* by H. Fletcher. Copyright 1953 by D. Van Nostrand Company, Inc. Reprinted by permission of Wadsworth Publishing Company, Belmont, California 94002.

intelligible speech. Hand-painted versions were produced by first drawing the most apparent features of the original, and then modifying the patterns while listening to the results until, usually by trial and error, the simplified drawn spectrograms were fairly intelligible. In the example shown in figure 7.6, both the original and the hand-painted versions could be used with the pattern playback to produce an understandable acoustic rendition of "to catch pink salmon." Pattern playback not only permits editing of sound spectrograms to determine which components are necessary for intelligibility, but also permits synthesis of acoustic patterns with desired characteristics.

In the early years of the sound spectrogram's use, it was hoped that it would provide a "visual speech" permitting the deaf to see and comprehend spoken language (see Potter, Kopp, & Kopp, 1947). However, sound spectrograms have proved disappointingly difficult to read, even with considerable training. One reason for this difficulty appears to be the interaction of phonemes in normal speech. The statement has been made by a scientist using spectrograms that "As a matter of fact I have not met one single speech researcher who has claimed he could read speech spectrograms fluently, and I am no exception myself" (Fant, 1962). Samples of single vowels produced in isolation or by careful choice of neighboring sounds in monosyllables (such as

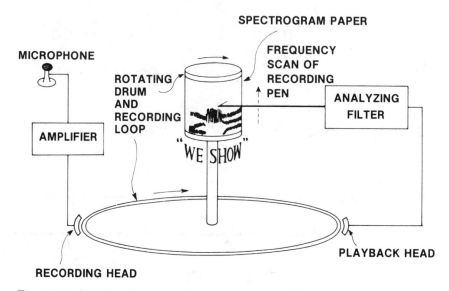

Fig. 7.5. Schematic diagram of the structure and functioning of the sound spectrograph, as available in models by Kay Elemetrics Co. and Voice Identification, Inc.
Source: J. M. Pickett, *The Sounds of Speech Communication: A Primer of Acoustic Phonetics and Speech Perception* (Baltimore, Md.: University Park Press, 1980.)

/h*d/, where * represents the vowel) can be characterized and identified relatively easily using spectrograms; but, in running speech, the boundaries between phonemes are often lost, and the acoustic nature of a speech sound is found to be influenced greatly by the nature of the neighboring sounds. The coarticulation effect of one speech sound upon another sometimes extends for a few phonemes before and after its occurrence. It has been suggested that such context-sensitive allophones (variants of the same phoneme) may enhance identification of the brief phonemic components of speech by providing information concerning more than one phoneme simultaneously (Wickelgren, 1969).

It is evident that coarticulation does not interfere with either comprehension of speech or the identification of constituent phonemes by listeners. Why, then, does coarticulation appear to make the reading of sound spectrograms so difficult? One possible explanation is that we have had many thousands of hours practice listening to speech, and a tremendous amount of practice in reading spectrograms is required before we can achieve comparable performance. In support of this explanation, fairly good performance (although still not matching auditory perception of speech) has been reported for an individual having an estimated 2,000 to 2,500 hours practice reading

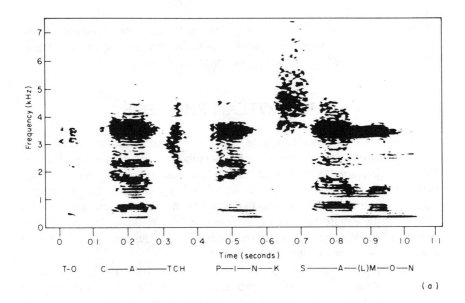

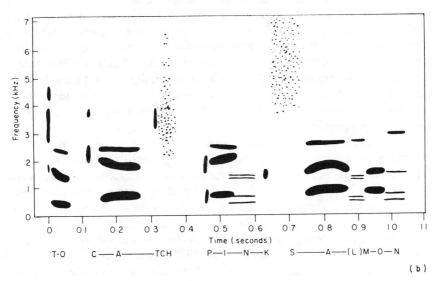

Fig. 7.6. (a) Sound spectrogram of a phrase; (b) Simplified version of the same phrase, painted by hand. Both of these versions are intelligible after conversion to sound by the "pattern playback" device.

Source: A.M. Liberman, P. Delattre, and F.S. Cooper, "The Role of Selected Stimulus-Variables in the Perception of the Unvoiced Stop Consonants," *American Journal of Psychology* 65 (1952): 497-516. Copyright 1952 by K. M. Dallenbach, reproduced by permission of The University of Illinois Press.

sound spectrograms (Cole, Rudnicky, Zue, & Reddy, 1980). However, it also is possible that sound spectrograms do not make visible some subtle acoustic characteristics used for auditory perception of speech.

THE PROTEAN PHONEME

As we have seen, a phoneme can assume different forms that are determined, to a great degree, by the identity of the neighboring speech sounds. This has led to what Klatt (1979) has called the "acoustic-phonetic non-invariance problem." If phonemes have a perceptual reality, they might be expected to possess some acoustic characteristics, or cluster of characteristics, which serve to differentiate one phoneme from another. However, despite careful searches for such phonetic invariance, it has not always been possible to find convincing evidence of its existence.

Individual plosive consonants are especially difficult to characterize in terms of acoustically invariant properties. They cannot be produced in isolation, and when articulated with a vowel to form a consonant-vowel syllable, sound spectrograms indicate that their acoustic forms are determined by adjacent vowels. Figure 7.7 shows spectrogram patterns which can be played back to produce syllables corresponding to /di/ and /du/. It can be seen that in /di/, the second formant rises from about 2,200 to 2,600 Hz, while in /du/ it falls from about 1,200 to 700 Hz. When the formant transitions are heard in isolation without the subsequent portion corresponding to the vowels, the frequency glides of the plosives resemble whistles or glissandos rather than speech sounds.

In the 1960s, there were attempts to save the acoustically elusive phoneme by considering it to be closely related to speech production. According to the motor theory of speech perception (Liberman, Cooper, Shankweiler, & Studdert-Kennedy, 1967), the afferent auditory signal is interpreted neurally in terms of the efferent motor commands necessary to produce the signal. Since acoustic invariance is not a necessary concomitant of motor invariance, the theory can handle the perceptual equivalence of different acoustic input. However, MacNeilage (1970) has presented evidence that electromyographic (muscle) recordings made during the production of phonemes in different contexts have indicated the absence of a motor invariance as well. Analysis-by-synthesis (Halle & Stevens, 1972; Stevens, 1960; Stevens & Halle, 1967) also considers a close relation between perception and mechanisms for speech production. It is considered that the auditory signal is subject to analysis in terms of features possessed by phonemes, such as those hypothesized in the linguistic feature systems of Chomsky and Halle (1968) or of Jakobson, Fant, and Halle (1963). This analysis permits generation of rules used for production of the sound. Hypotheses are then con-

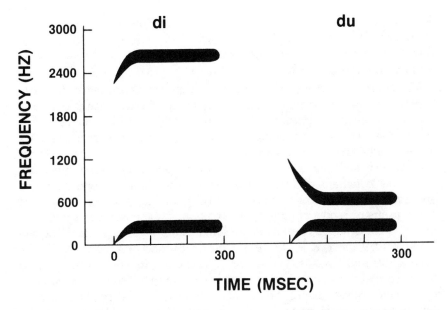

Fig. 7.7. Spectrographic patterns sufficient for the synthesis of /d/ before /i/
and before /u/ when converted to sound.
Source: From A.M. Liberman, F.S. Cooper, D.P. Shankweiler, and M. Stud-
    dert-Kennedy, "Perception of the Speech Code," *Psychological Re-
    view* 74 (1967): 431-61. Copyright 1967 by the American Psychologi-
    cal Association and reprinted by permission of the publisher and
    A.M. Liberman.

structed based on these generative rules, and these hypotheses are used to
construct an internal auditory pattern consisting of phonetic segments. This
internal pattern is compared with the pattern produced by the acoustic input,
and recognition results if the match is close. If the match is not close, new
hypotheses and new internal patterns are generated for comparison with the
patterns produced by the stimulus.

Both analysis-by-synthesis and the motor theory of speech perception
accept the existence of phonemes as perceptual entities, but do not require
them to have an acoustic invariance. However, starting in the 1970s there
have been several attempts to describe phonemes in terms of invariant
aspects. A number of investigators have suggested that, while many acoustic
characteristics of phonemes vary with context, certain cues (not always
apparent when looking at waveforms or spectrograms) are invariant and
used for phonemic identification (Cole & Scott, 1974; Jusczyk, Smith, &
Murphy, 1981; Searle, Jacobson, & Rayment, 1979; Stevens, 1971; Stevens
& Blumstein, 1981). While it appears that there are some acoustic characteristics which are invariant for some phonemes, it seems that definitive evi-

dence for acoustic invariance of other phonemes, particularly the plosive consonants, is not available at present. Diehl (1981) has gone so far as to suggest that some evidence cited as supporting an acoustic invariance model actually provides evidence against this model.

A different type of invariance has been proposed for phonemic identification based upon integrated responses from specialized neural analyzers operating as subphonemic feature detectors (Cooper, 1974; Eimas & Corbit, 1973). The difficulties encountered in specifying acoustic characteristics defining individual phonemes are met by considering identification of a phoneme to be based upon a set of characteristics analyzed by a set of hypothetical linguistic feature detectors. Claims of experimental support for this approach are based upon studies using "feature detector adaptation" in which listeners report apparent changes in a test stimulus occurring after repeated presentation of an adapting stimulus (for reviews of this work, see Cooper, 1979; Eimas & Miller, 1978; Simon & Studdert-Kennedy, 1978). The general rule found was that repetition caused category boundaries (such as the voice onset time boundary separating /t/ from /d/) to shift in the direction of the voice onset time of the repeated stimulus, and these changes were attributed to the adaptation of linguistic feature detectors. However, several recent investigators have suggested that the effects of repetition are the consequence of general effects of adaptation and fatigue applicable to both speech and nonspeech, so that there is no need to postulate the existence of specific linguistic feature detectors (see Diehl, 1981; Elman, 1979; Rosen, 1979; Sawusch & Nusbaum, 1979; Simon & Studdert-Kennedy, 1978).

Before proceeding further with mechanisms for speech perception, it is necessary to look more deeply into the role of the phoneme in speech perception. There can be little doubt that phonemes are extremely useful (and perhaps indispensable) constructs for the study of speech production and for linguistic analysis. However, as we have seen, perceptual models based on the recovery of phonemes from speech have run into difficulties, often attributable to the "acoustic-phonetic non-invariance problem."

ARE PHONEMES PERCEPTUAL UNITS?

The Alphabet and the Phoneme

Alphabetic writing originated as an attempt to specify individual speech sounds by letters and, hence, letters are related to modern phonetic symbols (see Gleitman & Rozin, 1977). Of course, modern English spelling differs considerably from modern English pronunciation; but it is still possible to try to pronounce an unfamiliar word from inspection of its written form with a fair chance of success. Those who believe that a phoneme is a natural unit of speech generally consider that the development of alphabetic writing represents the recognition of a fact of nature. But there are those who think otherwise; for example, Lüdtke (1969) has suggested that the alphabet is an artificial construct based upon "historical contingency," and that phonemic theory represents a consequence of this writing system. Lüdtke attributed the failure of experimental attempts to demonstrate the physical reality of phonemes to the artificial nature of the construct. There have been recent studies with both adults and children that have supported this view by showing that there is a close relation between literacy in alphabetic writing and the ability to identify phonemes.

Illiterate Adults Cannot Segment Phonetically

Morais, Cary, Alegria, and Bertelson (1979) tested adults of "peasant origin" living in a poor agricultural region of Portugal. Half of these adults were illiterate (Group I), and the other half had some familiarity with reading following attendance in special classes for illiterates (Group R). Both groups were required either to add the sounds [m], [p] or [ʃ] to an utterance produced by the experimenter, or to delete these sounds from a different set of utterances by the experimenter. It was found that Group I could neither delete nor add the designated speech sounds at the beginning of a nonsense word, while Group R had little difficulty with this task. Morais and his colleagues concluded that their results "...clearly indicate that the ability to deal explicitly with the phonetic units of speech is not acquired spontaneously. Learning to read, whether in childhood or as an adult, evidently allows the ability to manifest itself."

Ability to Segment Phonetically and Reading Ability Are Related in Children

Before learning to read, children can identify the number of syllables in a short utterance much better than they can the presence of an equal number of phonemes. Liberman, Shankweiler, Fischer, and Carter (1974) tested three groups of children in nursery school, kindergarten, and first grade (4-, 5-, and 6-year-olds) who listened to utterances containing one to three units (either syllables or phonemes depending on the "game"), and then indicated by the number of taps on a table how many units were present. Each age group performed much better at syllabic segmentation than phonetic segmentation. Only the children five and six years of age had been receiving instruction in reading; and it was found that while no children could segment phonetically at four years of age, 17 percent could segment at age five, and 48 percent at age six.

There have been a number of claims that children starting to read encounter considerable difficulty in the task of segmenting spoken words into sequences of discrete units, as required to appreciate the nature of alphabetic writing (Calfee, Chapman, & Venezky, 1972; Gibson & Levin, 1975; Gleitman & Rozin, 1973; Savin, 1972). Rozin, Poritsky, and Sotsky (1971) found that children in the second grade with reading disabilities made rapid progress in learning to read when ideographic characters representing entire English words were used rather than alphabetic writing. Rozin and his colleagues concluded that their study, together with other evidence, indicated that "...the alphabetic unit or phoneme is unnatural or at least highly suspect." Other investigators working with children demonstrating reading difficulties have noted that these children also encounter problems when presented with other tasks requiring phonetic segmentation. Thus, children with reading disabilities have difficulties in finding syllables that rhyme, and in learning to speak Pig Latin (which involves shifting the initial consonant cluster of a word to its end and adding the dipthong /ei/ (see Monroe, 1932; Savin, 1972).

Cues for Identifying Phonemes and Characterizing Letters

When analyzing speech and trying to catalog its constituent elements, sounds corresponding to particular articulatory positions of the tongue and lips form especially obvious constituents. The articulatory invariance of a particular stop consonant can be quite clear to an observer. Thus, all tokens of the phoneme /p/ involve stopping the flow of air at the lips. Additional information concerning voicing permits discrimination between /p/ and /b/, and characterizes the phoneme unambiguously. Phonemes defined by articulatory position are not subject to the acoustic-phonetic non-invariance problem; thus, variations in formant transitions when /p/ is followed by different vowels become irrelevant. Also, MacNeilage's observation that there is no invariance in muscle activity associated with production of individual stop consonants is not a problem, since the articulatory invariance represents the end point of muscle activity (lip closure), not the muscular activity needed to achieve this position.

However, not all articulatory positions corresponding to phoneme production are available for analysis. As pointed out by Helmholtz,

> we have no idea at all of the form and the movements of such exquisitely sensitive parts as our soft palate, our epiglottis and our larynx because we cannot see them without optical instruments and cannot easily touch them. ...

The extraordinarily varied and minute movements of the larynx teach us also, regarding relation between the act of volition and its effect, that what we are able to produce first and directly is not the innervation of a certain nerve or muscle, nor is it always a certain position of the movable parts of our bodies, but it is the first observable external effect. As far as we can ascertain by eye and hand the position of the parts of our bodies, this is the first observable effect with which the conscious intent in the act of volition is concerned. Whenever we cannot do this, as in the larynx and in the posterior parts of the mouth, the different modifications of voice, breathing, swallowing, etc., are these first effects. (Warren & Warren, 1968, p. 234).

Helmholtz's comments would lead us to expect that, when people profoundly deaf from an early age try to produce intelligible speech, they have the greatest difficulty in exercising control over their larynx and articulatory positions at the back of the mouth. In keeping with these expectations, Peterson (1946) has observed that the three major problems associated with quality of speech by the deaf are: pitch variations (under laryngeal control), breathiness (under laryngeal control), and nasality (under velar, or soft palate, control).

Vowels are usually more difficult to characterize in terms of articulatory position than consonants, and X-rays are sometimes needed to establish these positions. Historically, vowels were the last of the phonemes to be represented by symbols, being preceded by consonant-syllabic scripts (Gleitman & Rozin, 1977). Also, children acquiring reading skills find it more difficult to deal with vowels than consonants, and make a larger number of errors with the letters corresponding to vowels (Shankweiler & Liberman, 1972).

Evidence that Phonetic Constituents of Speech Are Not Identified Directly

There are two lines of experimental evidence indicating that listeners do not perceive phonemes in running speech directly, but that their presence is inferred following identification of larger units on the syllabic or word level. One of these lines is based upon the phonemic restoration effect, and the other upon the time required to identify components.

It has been reported that listeners cannot detect which speech sound is missing after listening to a recorded sentence in which a phoneme has been deleted and replaced by a cough or noise burst (Warren, 1970b; Warren & Warren, 1970). Identification of the absent phoneme is accomplished through linguistic context rather than cues provided by adjacent context-sensitive allophones, since the contextually appropriate phoneme is reported to be present when a contextually inappropriate phoneme from a mispronounced word in the sentence is deleted and replaced by noise (Warren & Sherman, 1974). Samuel (1981b) has reported that phonemic restoration is influenced by the rules governing clustering of phonemes within words, as well as the rules of syntax and semantic factors operating at the sentence level. We will return to the phonemic restoration effect later, but the point of special interest here is that the restored phonemes are indistinguishable from those phonemes present as acoustic components of the stimulus. It is suggested that both the "restored" phonemes and the "real" phonemes are inferred entities based upon a holistic recognition of acoustic patterns corresponding to syllables or words.

Savin and Bever (1970) measured the times required to identify phonemes and syllables. Their listeners were instructed to press a key as soon as they heard a given target in a sequence of nonsense syllables. The targets consisted of initial consonants, the vowel following the consonant, or the entire syllable. It was found that the time required to respond to the syllable target was less than for the phonemes within the syllable. They concluded that access to the syllable occurred first, and that identification of the phonemes followed the recognition of the syllable.

The experimental results reported by Savin and Bever were confirmed in a study carried out shortly before their work was published. This study was undertaken to test the hypothesis (based upon the phonemic restoration effect) that the identity of phonemes was inferred following prior identification of larger units (Warren, 1971). In addition to using lists of nonsense syllables as did Savin and Bever, English words, and words forming sentences also were used. The sentences were designed with different transitional probabilities of target words; and, as would be anticipated, a target word within a sentence which was more probable on the basis of prior context could be identified more quickly than a target word which was less probable. But the finding of interest to theory was that contextual cues which speeded up identification of a target word also speeded up identification of phonemes and phoneme clusters within the word to the same extent. Hence, the identification of words and their constituent phonemes appears to be a serial process with the higher level organization preceding the lower, rather than a case of parallel processing with identification of phonemes taking longer than words. Subsequent studies have confirmed the basic observation that identification of a syllable or word takes less time than identification of a constituent phoneme. (See Massaro, 1979, for a description of this work and a discussion of the implications for theory.)

THE TEMPORAL COURSE OF SPEECH PERCEPTION

Since humans function as both producers and receivers (perceivers) of speech, it has been tempting, and to some extent useful, to look for similarities and interdependence of these two modes of linguistic behavior. Certainly, when operating as speaker or listener we use the same lexicon and linguistic conventions. However, there are basic differences between the goals and strategies employed for production and perception. A major distinction is that the course of temporal organization is reversed for producing and for perceiving speech.

When producing speech, knowledge of what is to be said precedes (or should precede) vocalization. In extended discourse, the general plan of what is to be communicated may be formulated by the speaker several sentences in advance; and, by the time a particular sentence is started, its structure must be well organized if speech is to maintain fluency and intelligibility. When listening rather than speaking, the temporal nature of the task is quite different: processing obviously does not precede but rather follows production. The message received may be subject to perceptual errors and confusions resulting from environmental noises, unfamiliarity with the speaker's pronunciation and style, false expectations of the speaker's intent, unintentional ambiguities in what the speaker is saying, etc. It is not always possible or desirable to ask the speaker to repeat or clarify statements, and misunderstandings are not uncommon, as we all know. There is evidence that one important technique for minimizing errors in perception of speech involves delaying the perceptual organization of a word until several subsequent words have been received.

Skilled Storage and Delayed Perceptual Organization of Speech

Several investigators have noted that speech must be stored and perceptual decisions deferred if errors are to be minimized. Chistovich (1962) reported that many errors were made when her subjects were instructed to repeat speech heard through headphones as quickly as possible. She suggested that these mistakes reflected the temporal course of speech identification, with an appreciable delay in response time being needed for more accurate performance. Both Miller (1962) and Lieberman (1963) have emphasized that successful speech perception cannot proceed as a Markovian process, with perception occurring first on lower and then higher levels of organization. Processing of this nature does not benefit fully from the redundancy of the message and does not permit the correction of mistakes. Without the possibility of correction, an error would continue to provide incorrect context, producing still more errors until comprehension became blocked. This is the sort of difficulty which can be encountered by someone with less than complete mastery of a foreign language.

Bryan and Harter (1897, 1899) reported evidence concerning the importance of skilled storage in linguistic comprehension. They worked with expert telegraphers who they claimed had learned a "telegraphic language" similar to other languages. Complete mastery required several years of continual use, perhaps 10 years to achieve the speed and accuracy required for a press dispatcher. Skill in sending messages was achieved relatively quickly; it was the receiving of messages which was more difficult. When mastery in receiving was achieved, the receiver could work automatically with little conscious effort, often transcribing complex messages while thinking about something quite different. The story has been told that a telegrapher who transcribed the message that Lincoln had just been shot exhibited surprise when he overheard this news some time later.

An expert telegrapher usually delayed several words before transcribing the ongoing text in normal messages. When receiving messages transmitted in cipher or when receiving stock quotations, the lack of hierarchical organization and redundancy made the task much harder for experts. In recognition of this difficulty, the sender slowed down the transmittal rate, and the receiver decreased the number of words held in storage by following the text more closely in time. Thus, long storage was used only when the context permitted useful interactions between information received at different times.

Skilled storage similar to that reported for telegraphy has been observed for typewriting (Book, 1925), for reading aloud (Huey, 1968), and for tactile reading by the blind (Love, cited by Bryan & Harter, 1899; Moore & Bliss, 1975). It appears that storage with continuing processing and revision is employed quite generally for comprehension of linguistic input. Lashley (1951) gave a classic demonstration of the use of storage to correct errors in speech perception made evident by subsequent context. He first spoke of the process of *rapid writing* to an audience. Several sentences after creating a set for the word *writing*, Lashley spoke the sentence: "Rapid righting with his uninjured hand saved from loss the contents of the capsized canoe." He then noted that the context required for the proper interpretation of the sounds corresponding to *righting* were not activated for some three to five seconds after hearing the word.

Phonemic restorations appear to provide a technique for studying perceptual organization of verbal information held in short-term storage. The original studies dealing with phonemic restoration (Warren, 1970b; Warren & Obusek, 1971) employed the stimulus sentence: "The state governors met with their respective legi*latures convening in the capitol city" (* designates an extraneous sound, such as a cough or noise burst, replacing the phoneme). The restored speech sound in this sentence could be identified solely on the basis of prior context, with no need for storage of acoustic information. However, other observations have indicated that listeners can restore phonemes on the basis of subsequent context, and that it is possible to defer the restoration of an ambiguous word fragment for several words until context is provided which resolves the ambiguity (Sherman, 1971; Warren & Warren, 1970).

SPEECH ERRORS IN EVERYDAY LIFE

There is an old medical maxim that pathology represents normal function laid bare. Disorders and errors in speech perception may also provide a means of glimpsing the otherwise hidden mechanisms of normal function. This hope of enhancing understanding of normal processes may underlie the continued study of speech errors since the late nineteenth century.

Most collections of naturally occurring speech errors deal with spontaneous errors in production, or "slips of the tongue." These are difficult to gather since they occur relatively infrequently, except for individuals especially prone to make these errors, such as the Reverend Dr. W. A. Spooner, an Oxford don who was Warden of New College, Oxford from 1903 to 1924. His "spoonerisms" include such statements as "you hissed my mystery lecture" for "you missed my history lecture" and "tasted the whole worm" rather than "wasted the whole term." The first comprehensive collection of slips of the tongue was Meringer's compendium published in Vienna (Meringer & Mayer, 1895). Recent collections of English slips of the tongue have been gathered by Fromkin (1971) and Shattuck (1975). These errors have been used in attempts to understand the planning and execution of phrases and sentences (see Fromkin, 1973, 1980).

In addition to studies of production errors, there have been a few attempts to collect errors in speech perception that have been detected while listening to speech in everyday life (see Browman, 1980; Celce-Murcia, 1980; Garnes & Bond, 1980). Errors in perception are much more common than errors in production, but they are quite difficult to study systematically. Perceptual errors can be caused by a variety of factors including interference by extraneous sounds, anticipatory bias, an unfamiliar accent or dialect, as well as a speaker's poor pronunciation. Often, errors remain undetected and listeners are left with an incorrect interpretation of the message. Despite the difficulties in collecting listeners' errors and evaluating their causes, compendia of errors can provide a measure of the reliability and accuracy of verbal communication under particular conditions, and can point to factors liable to cause difficulties in perceiving speech.

In addition to the collection of perceptual errors under normal listening conditions, it is possible to induce errors in the laboratory. The use of repeated verbal stimuli provides a convenient way of initiating perceptual errors.

CHANGES IN SPEECH PERCEPTION
DURING STIMULUS REPETITION

The shifts in category boundaries of speech sounds following the termination of stimulus repetition have been discussed earlier. This section deals with changes in perception of speech which occur during stimulus repetition. As we shall see, illusory changes in what is heard provide information concerning mechanisms employed for the perceptual organization of normal speech.

Verbal Satiation

When a word is repeated over and over to oneself, a lapse in meaning occurs which has been called verbal satiation or semantic satiation. Titchener (1915, pp. 26-27) described the effect as follows: "Repeat aloud some word—the first that occurs to you; *house,* for instance—over and over again; presently the sound of the word becomes meaningless and blank; you are puzzled and a morsel frightened as you hear it." Many studies have been reported on this topic, with some authors claiming that, occasionally, alternate meanings for the word may be introduced. (For review, see Amster, 1964.) The loss of meaning of words with continued stimulation is not unique for hearing, and occurs with viewing of printed words (Don & Weld, 1924; Severance & Washburn, 1907). Indeed, the loss of perceptual organization with continued stimulation by an unchanging pattern appears to be a general phenomenon, and will be discussed further in chapter 8.

Verbal Summation

Early in his career, B.F. Skinner (1936) discovered that listeners organized a sequence of indistinct speech sounds repeated over and over into meaningful words and phrases. He used recordings consisting of iterated sequences of three to five vowels which, when played softly, initially were heard as three to five syllables of indistinct speech. With continued listening to the repeated sequence, subjects thought that they could understand what the voice was saying, and believed that their responses were generally accurate. They sometimes heard statements referring to themselves and their private affairs, which were handled in part by telling a subject that the recording was prepared especially for him or her. After the listener responded, the stimulus was turned off, and another recording of indistinct vowels was presented. As we shall see, had Skinner left this recording on, he would have found that illusory changes occurred in what the voice seemed to be saying, and he would have discovered verbal transformations more than 20 years before they were first reported.

Since the original meaningless sequence of indistinct phonemes appeared to become clearer with repetition, acquiring illusory phonemes and meanings, Skinner called this device the "verbal summator." He suggested that the verbal summator could be used as a projective test or, as he put it, "a sort of verbal inkblot," and it was used subsequently by others for this purpose. However, when viewers see the forms of objects in ink blots, they generally attribute details of the ink blot to particular parts of an imagined figure without hallucinating new contours.With the verbal summator, listeners believed that they heard absent speech sounds.

Verbal Transformations

In verbal satiation studies, loss of meaning occurs when a subject both articulates and hears a repeated word. Rather different perceptual effects occur when subjects do not produce the iterated word but, instead, listen to a loud and distinctly enunciated word repeated by a loop of recorded tape or by a recirculating digital delay line. Subjects listening passively are not restricted to the perception of an unchanging sequence of speech sounds as with self-repetition. Instead, a series of illusory changes are heard in what the voice seems to be saying quite clearly (Warren & Gregory, 1958). It is as if verbal satiation is followed by verbal summation into a new verbal organization. The new verbal form is itself subject to satiation, with the process of decay and reorganization continuing as long as the repeated stimulus is heard. These illusory changes, which have been called verbal transformations (Warren, 1961a), can involve great perceptual distortions of the clearly pronounced words. Illusory changes also occur if the repeated word is faint or indistinct (as with the verbal summator), but illusory changes of initially unclear words take place at a lower rate than with an initially intelligible stimulus.

The first detailed study of verbal transformations (Warren, 1961a) employed young adults (British naval ratings), who heard repeated monosyllabic words and short sentences. Illusory changes were heard with all stimuli. When listening to a monosyllabic word repeated twice a second for three minutes, the average young adult heard about 30 transitions (or changes in what was heard) involving about six different forms (or different words), with transitions not only involving forms reported for the first time, but sometimes returning to forms which had been heard previously. An example of the illusory changes heard for the bisyllabic stimulus "seashore" is given below.

(A voice with standard English pronunciation was employed, and the terminal /r/ was not pronounced.) All of the illusory changes reported by one subject during three minutes are listed in order of occurrence: "seashore, see-shove, seashore, she-saw, seesaw, see-shove, seashore, she-saw-seesaw, seashore, she-saw-seesaw, seashore, she-sawve, seashore-seesaw, she-saw, seashore, see-saw-saw, seashell." Another subject in this study listening to the monosyllabic word "right" reported: "ripe, right, white, white-light, right, right-light, ripe, right, ripe, bright-light, right, ripe, bright-light, right, bright-light." As a final example, a third subject listening to the stimulus "fill-up" experienced fewer changes and greater distortion than most subjects: "fill-up, clock, fill-up, build-up, true love, build, broad, lunch, fill-up." It can be noted that the changes from one form to the next are frequently phonetically complex, and sometimes suggest semantic linkages.

Profound age differences have been found for verbal transformations. Warren (1961b) reported that the aged heard many fewer transitions and forms than young adults. The study was then extended to four groups of children (5, 6, 8, and 10 years of age) using the same stimuli employed in the earlier study with adults (Warren & Warren, 1966). It was found that verbal transformations did not occur at the age of 5 years. At 6 years, half of the children heard verbal transformations; appearance was all-or-none, so that the 6 year olds heard either no verbal transformations, or heard them occurring at a rate corresponding to that of older children and young adults. By the age of 8, all subjects heard verbal transformations. The rate of illusory changes remained approximately constant from 8 years of age through young adulthood, and declined markedly for subjects over 60 years of age. The number of different forms reported during three minutes of listening behaved somewhat differently, and declined regularly with age. Children often heard extensive changes involving several phonemes in going from one form to the next. A sample of all forms reported by an 8 year old child listening to the nonsense syllable "flime" repeated twice a second for three minutes follows: "flime, crime, clime, like, oink, clime, flime, haw, flying, flime, crime, fly-um, flime, flyed, oink, flyed, fly-in, Clyde, fly-in, oink, wink, fly-in, I'm flying, flying, Clyde, flying, oink, flyed, I'm flying, flyed, I wink, flyed, aw-wenk-ah" (Warren & Warren, 1966). In addition to age differences in extent of changes in going from one perceptual form to the next, there were differences in the nature of the words reported, indicating that organizational rules change with age. Miller (1962) has pointed out that "...language must contain some natural coding units of finite length. But what these coding units are for an articulate human being still remains something of a mystery." Verbal transformations do not solve this mystery, but do offer some clues indicating that the size of the "coding units" used for linguistic grouping changes consistently with age.

From ages 6 to 10, nonsense words were reported frequently with phonemes occurring in orders not permitted in English: for example, starting a word wtih the cluster "sr" as in "srime." Organization of young adults appeared to be limited strictly by the rules governing phoneme clustering: that is, they reported nonsense words fairly frequently; but, with no exceptions, the phonemes were clustered according to the rules of English. Listeners over 60 years of age generally employed meaningful English words as their units of organization. When presented with the repeated nonsense syllable "flime," the aged heard it as a meaningful word (an interesting exception is an incorrect past participle "flyed," reported more frequently than the actual nonsense stimulus by the aged).

Warren (1968c) suggested that the reorganization of repeated words is related to the reorganization of connected discourse employed when a preliminary organization of speech sounds into words and phrases is not confirmed by subsequent context. If verbal transformations reflect skilled reorganizational processes, they should not appear in children until their language skills have attained a certain level. The requisite level seems to be reached normally by the age of 6 or 7. The decrease in the nature and rate of verbal transformations in the aged may be attributable to adaptive changes in processing strategy. It is well established that considerable difficulty is encountered by the aged with tasks involving the use of complex storage following intervening activity (Welford, 1958). In view of this difficulty, the optimal strategy for the aged might be to organize speech directly into English words, with very little use of reorganization based on stored information and, hence, very few verbal transformations.

We maintain a mastery of linguistic skills over the greater part of our life span. It appears that this proficiency may be maintained, not through preserving a fixed repertoire of processing mechanisms, but rather through adaptive changes. A sort of perceptual homeostasis might be achieved through the use of mechanisms appropriate to changes in functional capacity. (See chapter 8 for a discussion of evidence that the rules governing perceptual interpretation of sensory input are continually being evaluated for accuracy, and are revised when appropriate.) If this view concerning adaptive changes is correct, then accuracy in speech perception can be achieved through a variety of perceptual strategies, and it is wrong to assume a similarity in mechanisms from a similarity in performance.

It has been suggested that the verbal transformation effect and the phonemic restoration effect are linked, each being related to mechanisms employed normally for the resolution of ambiguities and correction of errors (Warren & Warren, 1970). Obusek and Warren (1973), acting on this suggestion, combined these two illusions by presenting a repeated word ("magistrate") with a portion deleted and replaced by noise. If illusory changes are indeed corrective, they would be expected to be directed to the phonemically restored segment. When the /s/ of "magistrate" was removed and replaced by a louder noise, 42 percent of the illusory changes involved the position corresponding to the deleted /s/, compared to 5 percent when a different group of subjects heard the intact word as the repeated stimulus. When the /s/ was deleted and replaced by silence rather than noise (so that phonemic restorations were inhibited), the lability of phonemes heard in this position was greater than with the intact word, but much less than that associated with the presence of noise: only 18 percent of the changes involved the position of the gap. When the noise was present, it was not possible for a listener to detect which phoneme corresponded to the noise bursts any more than with phonemic restorations of nonrepeated sentences (Warren, 1970b). Yet, it appears that, at some level of processing, the distinction between speech-based and noise-based organization was maintained, and the perceptual reorganization was directed to the portion lacking direct acoustic justification.

There have been a number of attempts to find phonetically based rules governing the perceptual reorganization of verbal transformations (Barnett, 1964; Clegg, 1971; Evans & Wilson, 1968; Goldstein & Lackner, 1974; Naeser & Lilly, 1970). The failure of these studies to agree on general rules, either in terms of phonemes or distinctive features within phonemes (see Warren, 1976a), suggests that perception may proceed along other lines. Since transformations frequently involve simultaneous changes in several phonemes, it appears evident that some of the rules governing organization are to be found at a level above that corresponding to the phoneme.

Verbal transformations of dichotic stimuli have been used to study the nature of neural analyzers used for speech perception (Warren, 1977b; Warren & Ackroff, 1976b). In one of the conditions described in these papers, the stimulus word "tress" with a repetition period of 492 msec was passed through a digital delay line with two delay taps, and the delay between the taps was adjusted so that the asynchrony of the outputs was exactly half the repetition period (246 msec). Listening was through a pair of headphones wired separately so that temporally dichotic but otherwise identical stimuli were heard in each ear. Neither ear could be considered as leading with the half-cycle delay, and there was a lateral symmetry in the nature of simultaneous contralateral input. Since the interaural asynchrony was a few hundred milliseconds, there was no possibility of binaural fusion (see chapter 2); and all listeners initially perceived the stimulus correctly on each side. The question of interest to theory was whether or not the same illusory changes would be heard simultaneously on the right and left. If the changes were identical and simultaneous, it would indicate that there was a sharing of a single set of neural linguistic analyzers. If independent changes were to occur at each ear, then it would indicate that two sets of functionally separate analyzers were used for the acoustically identical verbal stimuli.

It was found that for each of 20 subjects, the times at which changes occurred were uncorrelated at each ear. Also, the forms heard at the two sides were independent, so that while the stimulus word "tress" might be perceived accurately at one ear, a word as far removed phonetically as "commence" might be heard at the other. Additional unpublished work by Warren and Bashford demonstrated that independent changes of the same word were not limited to only two competing versions. Listeners were presented with three asynchronous versions of a single repeated word, each separated from the other two by exactly one-third of the word's duration. Two versions were monaural (one on the right, and one on the left), and one was diotic with its apparent location lying in the medial plane. Each of the five listeners heard the three versions of the word (right, left, and center) change independently, and hence each was using three functionally independent sets of verbal analyzers for the same stimulus.

These observations indicate a degree of equipotentiality for cortical units employed for speech analysis, so that if one set of analyzers is occupied with a particular task, others can be assembled for analyzing identical phonetic sequences, at least up to the level of the word.

EAR ADVANTAGES AND CORTICAL PROCESSING OF SPEECH

One of an individual's cortical hemispheres plays the major role in the perception and production of speech. There is considerable evidence that the left hemisphere is dominant for the overwhelming majority of right-handed people and for about two-thirds of the left-handed population. Data concerning the dominant hemisphere for speech is available from clinical evidence involving loss of speech functions following unilateral brain damage produced by penetrating wounds, tumors, and strokes. In addition, it is possible to cause a temporary loss of linguistic functions by injecting a barbituate directly into the carotid artery on one side (the Wada test). If the side of the injected carotid artery corresponds to that of the dominant hemisphere for speech, a temporary loss of speech function is observed. Information concerning the location of the speech areas can provide important preoperative information for a neurosurgeon.

Ear advantages have been observed in accuracy of identification when competing stimuli are presented to each side (for reviews, see Berlin & McNeil, 1976; Prohovnik, 1978). Typically, right ear advantages are observed for speech, and left ear advantages for music. There is some controversy concerning the basis for these ear advantages. One explanation offered is that a cortical asymmetry in processing is coupled with a transmission advantage (enhanced by dichotic competition) of contralateral over ipsilateral pathways from ear to cortex (Kimura, 1967). Other explanations have been offered in terms of laterally directed attention and reporting strategies

(Kinsbourne, 1970; Lazarus-Mainka & Hörmann, 1978). It also seems possible that lateral asymmetries in the efficiency of processing information within subcortical centers and nuclei (either intrinsically determined or under efferent control) may be involved in ear advantages.

PERCEPTION OF LINGUISTIC AND NONLINGUISTIC SEQUENCES

It seems reasonable to assume that if permuted orders of sounds in sequences can be discriminated (as is the case for speech), then listeners have the ability to identify the component sounds and their orders. However, as described in chapter 5, work reported in the 1970s indicated that this common-sense view is not valid. It has been shown that direct identification of components and their orders in sequences of nonverbal sounds (such as hisses, tones, and buzzes) or verbal sounds (sequences of vowels) requires sounds with longer durations than the average for phonemes in speech. However, experiments with nonlinguistic sounds have demonstrated that listeners can distinguish readily between permuted orders of brief sounds at item durations much too brief to permit direct identification of order or even direct identification of component sounds. Once sequences can be identified holistically, listeners can learn to recite the names of components and their orders by rote. These findings with nonlinguistic sounds are consistent with the experiments discussed earlier in the present chapter indicating that component phonemes and their orders are not perceived directly but are inferred following identification of supraphonemic linguistic patterns.

Holistic pattern recognition is not restricted to humans. Evidence discussed in chapter 5 indicates that monkeys, cats, and dolphins can distinguish between permuted orders of nonverbal sounds, recognizing the overall pattern rather than the individual components and their orders. In addition, a number of laboratories have successfully taught animals to distinguish between different samples of speech, and have reported similarities in discrimination by these animals and by humans. Dewson (1964) taught cats to distinguish between /i/ and /u/ whether spoken by a male or female voice. Warfield, Ruben, and Glackin (1966) taught cats to distinguish between the words "cat" and "bat," and reported that the limits of acoustic alteration of the words permitting discrimination were similar for cats and for humans. Kuhl and Miller (1978) used synthetic speech and showed that chinchillas can distinguish between /ta/ and /da/, /ka/ and /ga/, and /pa/ and /ba/. In another study using natural speech, Kuhl and Miller (1974) found that, following training, syllables containing /t/ or /d/ could be discriminated by chinchillas despite variations in talkers, the vowels following the plosives, and the intensities. Work with monkeys by Sinnott, Beecher, Moody, and Stebbins (1976) has shown that they are able to discriminate between acoustic correlates of the place of human articulation with /ba/ and /da/. These studies indicate the extent to which the phylogenetic development of speech exploited perceptual abilities common to several widely separated mammalian species (for further discussion, see Warren, 1976b).

8

The Relation of Hearing to Other Senses

Books on perception usually concentrate on a single modality (such as vision or hearing) or a subdivision of a modality (for example, color vision or speech perception). Even when an introductory book on perception deals with several modalities, it is generally subdivided into sections with little overlap. The few books treating the senses together as a single topic generally emphasize philosophy or epistemology (but see Gibson, 1966; Marks, 1978).

Yet the senses are not independent. Events in nature are often multidimensional in character, and stimulate more than one sensory system. An organism which optimizes its ability to interact appropriately with the environment is one which integrates relevant information across sensory systems.

MULTIMODAL PERCEPTION

While speech perception may appear at first to be strictly an auditory task, this is not quite true. Lip reading (or speech reading) can play an important subsidiary role. But before dealing further with this interaction of modalities in speech perception, let us consider cross-modality interactions involving senses which do not include hearing.

Interaction of Vision with Senses Other than Hearing

Depth perception in vision is based on a number of cues, including disparity of the images at the two retinae, and motion parallax. But, in addition to these cues transmitted by the optic nerve, there are proprioceptive ocular cues from the muscles producing accommodation (changes in the curvature of the lens necessary to produce a sharp image) and convergence (adjustment of the ocular axes so that the fixated object is imaged on each fovea). These cues originating in muscles are integrated with, and are indistinguishable from, the purely optical cues to depth. For a person perceiving an object at a particular distance, these muscle-sense cues are as fully visual as those providing information via the optic nerve.

Another example of visual interaction is afforded by the vestibulo-ocular reflex, which helps the viewer maintain visual fixation that might otherwise be lost during head movements. Receptors in the semicircular canals found in the inner ear signal rotary acceleration of the head, and this information is transmitted by the vestibular branch of the auditory nerve. Reflex eye movements are produced by this stimulation in a direction that compensates for the effects of head movements. When the vestibular and ocular systems are operating normally in a coordinated fashion, we are unaware of the contribution of vestibular input to the stability of our visual world.

Graybiel and his associates have studied the effect of vestibular information on visual perception in a quantitative fashion using the "oculogyral illusion." This illusion can be observed when a person is accelerated in a rotating chair while viewing a dim star-like pattern in an otherwise dark room, with the position of the visual pattern being fixed relative to the head of the subject. At very low acceleration rates which would be imperceptible with the eyes closed ($0.12°/sec^2$) the visual target appears to be displaced in the direction of acceleration (Graybiel, Kerr, & Bartley, 1948), so that the only way of detecting acceleration is through the effect of vestibular input on vision. It appears as if the information from the vestibular branch of the VIIIth nerve and the IInd (optic) nerve are integrated into a single percept, with vestibular contributions leading to effects interpreted as strictly visual.

Interesting effects are observed when conflicts are generated between information furnished by the vestibulo-auditory nerve and the optic nerve. If a person with closed eyes is spun rapidly (say at $180°/sec$) in a rotating chair for a few minutes and then brought to rest in a few seconds, disruption of visual perception by vestibular after-effects takes place when the eyes are opened. Involuntary eye movements which occur following the vestibular stimulation cause images of stationary objects to move continuously over the retina. This vestibulo-ocular reflex leads to illusory movement of the visual world, which is coupled sometimes with rather unpleasant feelings of vertigo and nausea. Yet, ice-skaters do not experience such after-effects following very rapid rotation and a sudden stop from a practiced spin. The vestibulo-ocular reflex and illusory motion can not only be suppressed by appropriate training, but it also can be changed in direction. It has been reported that, after several weeks of continuous wearing of goggles which were fitted with prisms reversing right and left, the direction of the vestibulo-ocular reflex was reversed, so that rotary acceleration produced eye movements which could compensate for the effect of head movement upon the retinal image as seen through the prisms (Gonshor & Jones, 1973).

While vision appears to be dominant in cross-modality integration with vestibular information, vision does not exhibit dominance when it interacts with auditory information in the perception of speech.

Interaction of Vision and Hearing in Speech Perception

Research in the last few years has indicated that people with normal hearing use speech reading (lip reading) to a greater extent than had been realized previously. Visual information concerning what is being said seems to be heard rather than seen; that is, it enters into determining what we believe we hear the speaker say.

Comprehension based on speech reading alone is very difficult, although some deaf people can understand what a speaker is saying through close visual observation. While lip movements are considered the most important cues, some articulatory information may be furnished by movements of the jaw and Adam's apple. In addition, there are a variety of facial expressions and other gestures correlated with meaning but not related directly to articulation. Nevertheless, speech reading, at best, provides incomplete and ambiguous information concerning articulation. Some speech sounds are produced by articulatory movements which cannot be seen (for example, /h/ and /k/), and some sounds with articulatory movements which can be seen have "homophenes" with the same appearance (/m/, /p/, and /b/ involve similar lip movements, so that "may," "pay," and "bay" all look alike).

Recent experiments have indicated that speech reading can function not only as an alternative mode for perceiving speech by the deaf, but that visual cues to articulation provide a supplementary source of information used by people with normal hearing to enchance intelligibility under noisy environmental conditions (for example, see Dodd, 1977, 1980). Speech reading can be facilitated even by an auditory signal which is itself completely unintelligible. Rosen, Fourcin, and Moore (1981) used listeners with normal hearing and compared their ability to perceive what a speaker said using speech reading alone and speech reading supplemented with acoustic input corresponding to the fundamental frequency pattern of the speaker's voice. While the voice-pitch information by itself was unintelligible, it was found to produce a dramatic increase in the ability to understand what the speaker was saying when used in conjunction with speech reading.

Perceptual Resolution of Conflicting Visual and Auditory Information Concerning Speech

An interesting interaction occurs when visual and auditory information to speech are placed in conflict. McGurk and MacDonald (1976) in a paper entitled "Hearing Lips and Seeing Voices," used a video recording of a talker producing a consonant-vowel syllable while a dubbed sound tract showed production of a different consonant-vowel syllable. For example, when the sound of *ba-ba* was dubbed onto a video recording of *ga-ga*, 98 percent of adults and 80 percent of preschool children reported hearing *da-da*. It should be noted that there was not any awareness of a visual contribution to perception—listeners believed that the illusory *da-da* was heard and was solely auditory. The illusion occurred even with the knowledge of the nature of the visual and auditory input, and by closing their eyes, subjects could hear *ba-ba* which reverted to *da-da* when their eyes were opened. It is as if the modality serving as the source of the information were irrelevant to the perceptual task of determining the nature of the acoustic utterance, and so is not perceived directly.

A conflict between vision and hearing in speech perception leads to the pooling of cues and the "hearing" of visual information, but this type of conflict resolution does not take place with other tasks in which vision is pitted against hearing. When visual and auditory cues to the localization of a source are in disagreement, vision tends to dominate, and the sound usually is heard to come from the position close to that indicated by vision (see Bertelson and Radeau, 1981).

AUDITORY INPUT PERCEIVED AS TOUCH

An interesting example of an inability to determine the modality furnishing perceptual information is provided by "facial vision" of the blind. Obstacles can be avoided by some sightless people through echoes reflected from surfaces, yet they usually are unaware that they are using hearing, and frequently attribute the detection of obstacles to sensitivity of their face and forehead. Acoustic cues are perceived by them as "pressure waves" stimulating their skin, producing a sensation which gets stronger and assumes an unpleasant quality if they continue on a collision course (see Supa, Cotzin, & Dallenbach, 1944; Worchel & Dallenbach, 1947). Indeed, if the blind do not heed the auditory information indicating their approach to an obstacle, they might suffer actual injury to the head.

The inability of the blind to appreciate that hearing serves as the basis for their obstacle sense and their false perception of auditory input as tactile stimulation seem anomalous only if we consider that people can appreciate directly the nature of sensory input used for perceptual evaluation. However, this misattribution is consistent with the hypothesis that we are aware of events correlated with sensory input rather than sensation per se.

MULTIMODAL SENSORY CONTROL
OF SPEECH PRODUCTION

The level of our vocal output is monitored not only by hearing, but also by nonauditory information including "vocal effort" as signified by propriocep-tive feedback from the muscles involved in controlling subglottal pressure and laryngeal pulsing (see chapter 7), and tactile cues to the magnitude of vibration along the vocal tract. Normally, these cues are in agreement, and each supplements and confirms the information provided by the others. Interesting effects occur when unusual conflicts are introduced (as will be discussed shortly). However, blocking, or at least partial blocking, of one of the monitoring systems (such as the masking of auditory feedback by noise) does not produce the interference associated with conflicting cues, since other monitoring systems can be used to maintain normal functioning.

This multimodal information concerning the level of our voice alone is insufficient to allow us to speak at an appropriate intensity. It is inappropriate to speak softly to someone far away, and a listener might show annoyance were we to shout in his ear. It would be unsuitable to use the same vocal level speaking to someone at a cocktail party that we would use when speaking to someone at the same distance in a quiet room. We take these factors into account automatically when speaking. Thus, it has been demonstrated that we are quite familiar with the effects of the inverse square law, and that we can adjust the level of our voice to compensate quite accurately for intensity changes at the listener's position due to the distance our voice must carry to reach its target (Warren, 1968a; see chapter 4). Visual cues play an important role in estimating this distance.

In addition to using hearing to monitor our own vocal level, we also use hearing to evaluate the ambient noise level. The increase in vocal intensity accompanying an increase in background noise is called the Lombard reflex, and it helps ensure that we can be heard by our targeted listeners. It is only after the distance to the target listener and the ambient noise level are determined, that the intensity required for comprehension by the listener can be reckoned and compared with the feedback from the several sensory systems monitoring our own voice.

GENERAL PERCEPTUAL RULES AND
MODALITY-SPECIFIC RULES

The close interrelation of senses might lead us to believe that rules governing perception in one modality would apply to others as well. While it does seem that such general rules do exist, attempts to apply broad principles either across modalities or to different tasks within single modalities should be carried out with considerable caution.

The physical correlate theory is a case in point. As discussed in chapter 4, this theory considers that attempts to measure sensory intensity directly produce responses based on estimates of physical magnitudes. However, this general rule cannot tell us which physical magnitude serves as the correlate of intensity judgments involving a particular sensory system without detailed knowledge of that modality and the way it is used normally to evaluate stimulus relations.

Premature analogies across senses can inhibit the understanding of phenomena. An example is furnished by the perceptual transformations experienced in both hearing and vision with prolonged stimulation by a fixed pattern. During visual inspection of a two-dimensional ambiguous figure, such as an outline drawing of a cube, perception of the figure can flip from one perspective interpretation to another. It is tempting to consider that illusory changes in repeated words (see chapter 7) represent an auditory analog of visual reversible figures, and it appears that Warren and Gregory (1958) were led astray by this analogy. Evans (see Warren, 1981b) considered that these verbal transformations were an auditory analog of illusory changes experienced with stabilized retinal images (that is, images seen without the normal changes in retinal stimulation accompanying our ever-present eye movements), and he too may have been misled by an inappropriate analogy. Warren (1981b) has suggested that change in perceptual organization during continued stimulation represents a general perceptual phenomenon operating across modalities, but that the nature of perceptual reorganization reflects special strategies for perception which differ across modalities, with different strategies being used even for different classes of tasks within a single modality. Thus, it has been hypothesized that verbal transformations represent highly specialized reorganizational strategies employed in speech perception, and that repeating nonverbal auditory patterns are not subject to analogous changes (see chapter 7).

PERCEPTUAL CALIBRATION OF SENSORY INPUT

Verbal transformations and illusory changes in unchanging visual displays occur *during* a continued exposure to the same stimulus. There are other perceptual changes which can be measured *following* exposure to a stimulus. These poststimulation changes follow a consistent rule applying to many types of judgments involving different sensory modalities. The rule can be stated as follows: the perceptual classification of a stimulus occupying a position along a continuum is shifted following exposure to an exemplar occupying a different position along the continuum, so that judgmental boundaries move toward the value represented by the exemplar. Let us clarify this "perceptual recalibration" rule by examples.

Perceptual recalibration can be observed for speech perception. As discussed in chapter 7, the time separating plosive release of air and the onset of voicing can determine whether a syllable is heard as /ta/ or /da/. The voice onset time corresponding to this category boundary shifts noticeably following listening to either /ta/ or /da/ restated several times. Thus, after listening to exemplars of /ta/, the category boundary moves into what previously was the /ta/ domain, and a sample which had been at the category boundary is now clearly heard as /da/. It is not necessary to use category boundaries separating phonemes to observe such perceptual shifts. Remez (1979) reported that the perceptual boundary for a vowel in a continuum extending from the vowel to a nonspeech buzz could be changed in an analogous fashion by exposure to an exemplar at one end of the continuum. Similar effects of prior stimulation were described for judgments along a variety of visual continua by Gibson, one such continuum being that of visual curvature. Gibson observed that if a curved line convex to the left was examined for some time, a line presented subsequently had to be curved in the same direction to appear straight, and an objectively straight line appeared convex to the right. Gibson called this phenomenon "adaptation with negative after-effect," and described it in terms of the following general rule: "If a sensory process which has an opposite is made to persist by a constant application of its appropriate stimulus-conditions, the quality will diminish in the direction of becoming neutral, and therewith the quality evoked by any stimulus for the dimension in question will be shifted temporarily toward the opposite or complementary quality" (Gibson, 1937). Similar errors in judgment were cataloged for a number of after-effects of seen motion by Wohlgemuth (1911), who reported that the visual input corresponding to perception of a stationary display was subject to temporary recalibration in the direction of previously perceived movement. Thus, after viewing a moving display, a new display must move slightly in the direction previously seen in order to appear stationary, so that an objectively stationary display is seen to move in the opposite direction. Related observations with other perceptual continua were described in 1910 by von Kries (1962, p. 239) who attributed these errors to what he called "the law of contrast." Cathcart and Dawşon (1928, 1929) also discovered this rule governing perceptual shifts. They recognized its very broad applicability, naming it the "diabatic" effect. Helson (1964) tried to quantify this general principle with his "adaptation level theory," but this theory has had a rather limited success. There have been attempts to explain perceptual shifts produced by prior stimulation in terms of the adaptation of hypothetical neural feature detectors, but this approach, at least applied to phoneme boundary shifts, has come under considerable criticism (see chapter 7).

Perhaps these perceptual after-effects reflect a relativistic basis for judgments, with the criteria used for perceptual evaluation constructed from past exemplars in such a way that higher weighting is assigned to recent exemplars. Thus, it may not be necessary that neural adaptation or fatigue take place for perceptual judgments to change. A shift or recalibration of criteria used for evaluation could be responsible for judgmental shifts. In keeping with this model, it can be considered that a consistent change in sensory patterning maintained for brief periods leads to perceptual recalibration with temporary "after-effects" upon return to the previous norm as described above, while extended exposure to alteration in sensory input leads to the adoption of more permanent perceptual norms consistent with the new conditions. (See the discussion of adjustment to the spatial rearrangement produced by "pseudophones" in chapter 2.)

There is evidence that "sensory deprivation" or absence of patterned sensory input can lead to a breakdown in normal perceptual processing (see Riesen, 1975; Schultz, 1965; Vernon, 1963). When subjects see only a featureless white field through translucent goggles and hear only white noise, disorientation along with visual and auditory hallucinations occur within a short time. After a few hours of such sensory deprivation, subjects experience errors in perceptual evaluation when returned to a normal environment. Perhaps calibration of sensory input occurs continuously, and is required to maintain appropriate perceptual interpretation of environmental events.

References

Abbagnaro, L. A., Bauer, B. B., & Torick, E. L. Measurements of diffraction and inter-aural delay of a progressive sound wave caused by the human head-II. *Journal of the Acoustical Society of America*, 1975, **58**, 693-700.

Adrian, E. D. The microphonic action of the cochlea: An interpretation of Wever and Bray's experiments. *Journal of Physiology*, 1931, **71**, 28-29.

Amster, H. Semantic satiation and generation: Learning? Adaptation? *Psychological Bulletin*, 1964, **62**, 273-286.

Bachem, A. Chroma fixation at the ends of the musical frequency scale. *Journal of the Acoustical Society of America*, 1948, **20**, 704-705.

Barnett, M. R. *Perceived phonetic changes in verbal transformation effect*. Doctoral dissertation, Ohio University, 1964.

Bashford, J. A., Jr., & Warren, R. M. Perceptual synthesis of deleted phonemes. In J. J. Wolf and D. H. Klatt (Eds.), *Speech Communication Papers*. New York: Acoustical Society of America, 1979, 423-426.

Batteau, D. W. The role of the pinna in human localizaton. *Proceedings of the Royal Society (London)*, Series B, 1967, **168**, 158-180.

Batteau, D. W. Listening with the naked ear. In S. J. Freedman (Ed.), *Neuropsychology of Spatially Oriented Behavior*. Homewood, Ill.: Dorsey Press, 1968, 109-133.

Békésy, G. von. Ueber die Entstehung der Entfernungsempfindung beim Hören, *Akustische Zeitung*, 1938, **3**, 21-31.

Békésy, G. von. Similarities between hearing and skin sensation. *Psychological Review*, 1959, **66**, 1-22.

Békésy, G. von. *Experiments in hearing*. New York: McGraw-Hill, 1960.

Bergman, M. Binaural hearing. *Archives of Otolaryngology*, 1957, **66**, 572-578.

Berlin, C. I., & McNeil, M. R. Dichotic listening. In N. J. Lass (Ed.), *Contemporary issues in experimental phonetics*. New York: Academic Press, 1976, 327-387.

Bertelson, P., & Radeau, M. Cross-modal bias and perceptual fusion with auditory-visual spatial discordance. *Perception & Psychophysics*, 1981, **29**, 578-584.

Bezold, W. von. Urteilstauschungen nach Beseitigung einseitiger Harthörigkeit. *Zeitschrift für Psychologie*, 1890, **1**, 486-487.

Bilsen, F. A. Repetition pitch: Its implication for hearing theory and room acoustics. In R. Plomp and G. F. Smoorenburg (Eds.), *Frequency analysis and periodicity detection in hearing.* Leiden, The Netherlands: Sijthoff, 1970, 291-302.

Bilsen, F. A. Pitch of noise signals: Evidence for a "central spectrum." *Journal of the Acoustical Society of America,* 1977, **61,** 150-161.

Bilsen, F. A., & Goldstein, J. L. Pitch of dichotically delayed noise and its possible spectral basis. *Journal of the Acoustical Society of America,* 1974, **55,** 292-296.

Bilsen, F. A., & Ritsma, R. J. Repetition pitch and its implication for hearing theory. *Acustica,* 1969/70, **22,** 63-73.

Bilsen, F. A., & Ritsma, R. J. Some parameters influencing the perceptibility of pitch. *Journal of the Acoustical Society of America,* 1970, **47,** 469-475.

Blauert, J. Sound localization in the median plane. *Acustica,* 1969/70, **22,** 205-213.

Bloch, E. Das binaurale Hören. *Zeitschrift für Ohrenheilkunde,* 1893, **24,** 25-85.

Blodgett, H. C., Wilbanks, W. A., & Jeffress, L. A. Effects of large interaural differences upon the judgment of sidedness. *Journal of the Acoustical Society of America,* 1956, **28,** 639-643.

Boer, E. de. On the "residue" in hearing. Doctoral dissertation, University of Amsterdam, 1956.

Boer, E. de. On the "residue" and auditory pitch perception. In W.D. Keidel and W.D. Neff (Eds.), *Handbook of sensory physiology,* Vol.V. *Auditory system.* Part 3: *Clinical and special topics.* Berlin: Springer-Verlag, 1976, 479-583.

Bond, Z. S. On the specification of input units in speech perception. *Brain & Language,* 1976, **3,** 72-87.

Book, W. F. *The psychology of skill with special reference to its acquisition in typewriting.* New York: Gregg, 1925.

Boring, E. G. *Sensation and perception in the history of experimental psychology.* New York: Appleton-Century-Crofts, 1942.

Bouhuys, A. Airflow control by auditory feedback: Respiratory mechanics and wind instruments. *Science,* 1966, **154,** 797-799.

Bregman, A. S., & Campbell, J. Primary auditory stream segregation and perception of order in rapid sequences of tones. *Journal of Experimental Psychology,* 1971, **89,** 244-249.

Bregman, A. S., & Dannenbring, G. L. Auditory continuity and amplitude edges. *Canadian Journal of Psychology,* 1977, **31,** 151-159.

Broadbent, D. E., & Ladefoged, P. Auditory perception of temporal order. *Journal of the Acoustical Society of America,* 1959, **31,** 1539-1540.

Brookshire, R. H. Visual and auditory sequencing by aphasic subjects. *Journal of Communication Disorders,* 1972, **5,** 259-269.

Browman, C. P. Perceptual processing: Evidence from slips of the ear. In V. A. Fromkin (Ed.), *Errors in linguistic performance: Slips of the tongue, ear, pen, and hand.* New York: Academic Press, 1980, 213-230.

Brown, E. L., & Deffenbacher, K. *Perception and the senses.* New York: Oxford University Press, 1979.

Bryan, W. L., & Harter, N. Studies in the physiology and psychology of the telegraphic language. *Psychological Review,* 1897, **4,** 27-53.

Bryan, W. L., & Harter, N. Studies on the telegraphic language: The acquisition of a hierarchy of habits. *Psychological Review,* 1899, **6,** 345-375.

Bukofzer, M. F. *Music in the baroque era.* New York: Norton, 1947.

Butler, R. A. Monaural and binaural localization of noise bursts vertically in the median sagittal plane. *Journal of Auditory Research,* 1969, **3**, 230-235.

Butler, R. A., Levy, E. T., & Neff, W. D. Apparent distance of sounds recorded in echoic and anechoic chambers. *Journal of Experimental Psychology: Human Perception and Performance,* 1980, **6**, 745-750.

Butler, R. A., & Naunton, R. F. Some effects of unilateral auditory masking upon the localization of sound in space. *Journal of the Acoustical Society of America,* 1962, **34**, 1100-1107.

Butler, R. A., & Naunton, R. F. Role of stimulus frequency and duration in the phenomenon of localization shifts. *Journal of the Acoustical Society of America,* 1964, **36**, 917-922.

Calfee, R., Chapman, R., & Venezky, R. How a child needs to think to learn to read. In L. W. Gregg (Ed.), *Cognition in learning and memory.* New York: Wiley, 1972, 139-182.

Carmon, A., & Nachshon, I. Effect of unilateral brain damage on perception of temporal order. *Cortex,* 1971, **7**, 410-418.

Cathcart, E. P., & Dawson, S. Persistence: A Characteristic of remembering. *British Journal of Psychology,* 1928, **18**, 262-275.

Cathcart, E. P., & Dawson, S. Persistence (2). *British Journal of Psychology,* 1929, **19**, 343-356.

Celce-Murcia, M. On Meringer's corpus of "slips of the ear." In V. A. Fromkin (Ed.), *Errors in linguistic performances: Slips of the tongue, ear, pen, and hand.* New York: Academic Press, 1980, 199-211.

Cherry, C., & Wiley, R. Speech communications in very noisy environments. *Nature,* 1967, **214**, 1164.

Chistovich, L. A. Temporal course of speech sound perception. In *Proceedings of the 4th International Commission on Acoustics* (Article H 18). Copenhagen: 1962.

Chocholle, R., & Legouix, J. P. On the inadequacy of the method of beats as a measure of aural harmonics. *Journal of the Acoustical Society of America,* 1957, **29**, 749-750. (a)

Chocholle, R., & Legouix, J. P. About the sensation of beats between two tones whose frequencies are nearly in a simple ratio. *Journal of the Acoustical Society of America,* 1957, **29**, 750. (b)

Chomsky, N., & Halle, M. *The sound patterns of English.* New York: Harper & Row, 1968.

Clegg, J. M. Verbal transformations on repeated listening to some English consonants. *British Journal of Psychology,* 1971, **62**, 303-309.

Colavita, F. B., Szeligo, F. V., & Zimmer, S. D. Temporal patten discrimination in cats with insular-temporal lesions. *Brain Research,* 1974, **79**, 153-156.

Cole, R. A., Rudnicky, A. I., Zue, V. W., & Reddy, D. R. Speech as patterns on paper. In R. A. Cole (Ed.), *Perception and production of fluent speech.* Hillsdale, N.J.: Erlbaum, 1980, 3-50.

Cole, R. A., & Scott, B. Perception of temporal order in speech: The role of vowel transitions. *Canadian Journal of Psychology,* 1973, **27**, 441-449.

Cole, R.A., & Scott, B. The phantom in the phoneme: Invariant cues for stop consonants. *Perception & Psychophysics,* 1974, **15**, 101-107.

Coleman, P. D. An analysis of cues to auditory depth perception in free space. *Psychological Bulletin*, 1963, **60**, 302-315.

Cooper, W. E. Contingent feature analysis in speech perception. *Perception & Psychophysics*, 1974, **16**, 201-204.

Cooper, W. E. *Speech perception and production: Studies in selective adaptation.* Norwood, N.J.: Ablex, 1979.

Cramer, E. M., & Huggins, W. H. Creation of pitch through binaural interaction. *Journal of the Acoustical Society of America*, 1958, **30**, 413-417.

Cullinan, W. L., Erdos, E., Schaefer, R., & Tekieli, M. E. Perception of temporal order of vowels and consonant-vowel syllables. *Journal of Speech and Hearing Research*, 1977, **20**, 742-751.

Dallos, P. *The auditory periphery: Biophysics and physiology.* New York: Academic Press, 1973.

Dallos, P. Biophysics of the cochlea. In E. C. Carterette and M. P. Freedman (Eds.), *Handbook of perception*, Vol. 4. New York: Academic Press, 1978, 125-162.

Dallos, P. Cochlear physiology. *Annual Review of Psychology*, 1981, **32**, 153-190.

Dannenbring, G. L. Perceived auditory continuity with alternately rising and falling frequency transitions. *Canadian Journal of Psychology*, 1976, **30**, 99-114.

David, E. E., Guttman, N., & van Bergeijk, W. A. On the mechanism of binaural fusion. *Journal of the Acoustical Society of America*, 1958, **30**, 801-802.

Davis, H. Some principles of sensory receptor action. *Physiological Review*, 1961, **41**, 391-416.

Davis, H. A model for transducer action in the cochlea. *Cold Spring Harbor Symposium on Quantitative Biology*, 1965, **30**, 181-190.

Davis, H. Discussion of Batteau's contribution. In A. V. S. de Reuck and J. Knight (Eds.), *Hearing mechanisms in vertebrates, CIBA foundation symposium.* Boston: Little, Brown, 1968, 241-242.

Davis, H., Benson, R. W., Covell, W. P., Fernandez, C., Goldstein, R., Katsuki, Y., Legouix, J.-P., McAuliffe, D. R., & Tasaki, I. Acoustic trauma in the guinea pig. *Journal of the Acoustical Society of America*, 1953, **25**, 1180-1189.

Davis, H., Fernandez, C., & McAuliffe, D. R. The excitatory process in the cochlea. *Proceedings of the National Academy of Sciences* (U.S.A.), 1950, **36**, 580-587.

Deinse, J. B. van. Registers. *Folia Phoniatrica*, 1981, **33**, 37-50.

Del Castillo, D. M., & Gumenik, W. E. Sequential memory for familiar and unfamiliar forms. *Journal of Experimental Psychology*, 1972, **95**, 90-96.

Deutsch, D. An auditory illusion. *Nature*, 1974, **251**, 307-309.

Deutsch, D. Two-channel listening to musical scales. *Journal of the Acoustical Society of America*, 1975, **57**, 1156-1160.

Deutsch, D. The octave illusion and auditory perceptual integration. In J. V .Tobias and E. D. Schubert (Eds.), *Hearing research and theory*, Vol.1. New York: Academic Press, 1981, 99-142.

Deutsch, D., & Roll, P. L. Separate "what" and "where" decision mechanisms in processing a dichotic tonal sequence. *Journal of Experimental Psychology: Human Perception and Performance*, 1976, **2**, 23-29.

Dewson, J. H. III. Speech sound discrimination by cats. *Science*, 1964, **144**, 555-556.

Dewson, J. H. III, & Cowey, A. Discrimination of auditory sequences by monkeys. *Nature*, 1969, **222**, 695-697.

Diehl, R. L. Feature detectors for speech: A critical reappraisal. *Psychological Bulletin*, 1981, **89**, 1-18.

Dirks, D. D., & Bower, D. Effect of forward and backward masking on speech intelligibility. *Journal of the Acoustical Society of America*, 1970, **47**, 1003-1008.

Divenyi, P. L., & Hirsh, I. J. Identification of temporal order in three-tone sequences. *Journal of the Acoustical Society of America*, 1974, **56**, 144-151.

Dodd, B. The role of vision in the perception of speech. *Perception*, 1977, **6**, 31-40.

Dodd, B. Interaction of auditory and visual information in speech perception. *British Journal of Psychology*, 1980, **71**, 541-549.

Don, V. J., & Weld, H. P. Minor studies from the psychological laboratory of Cornell University. LXX. Lapse of meaning with visual fixation. *American Journal of Psychology*, 1924, **35**, 446-450.

Dorman, M. F., Cutting, J. E., & Raphael, L. J. Perception of temporal order in vowel sequences with and without formant transitions. *Journal of Experimental Psychology: Human Perception and Performance*, 1975, **104**, 121-129.

Dowling, W. J. The perception of interleaved melodies. *Cognitive Psychology*, 1973, **5**, 322-337.

Efron, R. Temporal perception, aphasia, and déjà vu. *Brain*, 1963, **86**, 403-424.

Efron, R. Conservation of temporal information by perceptual systems. *Perception & Psychophysics*, 1973, **14**, 518-530.

Efron, R., & Yund, E. W. Ear dominance and intensity independence in the perception of dichotic chords. *Journal of the Acoustical Society of America*, 1976, **59**, 889-898.

Egan, J. P. The effect of noise in one ear upon the loudness of speech in the other. *Journal of the Acoustical Society of America*, 1948, **20**, 58-62.

Egan, J. P., & Hake, H. W. On the masking pattern of a simple auditory stimulus. *Journal of the Acoustical Society of America*, 1950, **20**, 622-630.

Eimas, P. D., & Corbit, J. D. Selective adaptation of linguistic feature detectors. *Cognitive Psychology*, 1973, **4**, 99-109.

Eimas, P. D., & Miller, J. L. Effects of selective adaptation on the perception of speech and visual patterns: Evidence for feature detectors. In R. D. Walk and H. L. Pick (Eds.), *Perception and experience*. New York: Plenum, 1978, 307-345.

Elfner, L. F. Continuity in alternately sounded tone and noise signals in a free field. *Journal of the Acoustical Society of America*, 1969, **46**, 914-917.

Elfner, L. F. Continuity in alternately sounded tonal signals in a free field. *Journal of the Acoustical Society of America*, 1971, **49**, 447-449.

Elfner, L. F., & Caskey, W. E. Continuity effects with alternately sounded noise and tone signals as a function of manner of presentation. *Journal of the Acoustical Society of America*, 1965, **38**, 543-547.

Elfner, L. F., & Homick, J. L. Some factors affecting the perception of continuity in alternately sounded tone and noise signals. *Journal of the Acoustical Society of America*, 1966, **40**, 27-31.

Elfner, L. F., & Homick, J. L. Continuity effects with alternately sounding tones under dichotic presentation. *Perception & Psychophysics*, 1967, **2**, 34-36. (a)

Elfner, L. F., & Homick, J. L. Auditory continuity effects as a function of the duration and temporal location of the interpolated signal. *Journal of the Acoustical Society of America*, 1967, **42**, 576-579. (b)

Elliot, L. L. Backward and forward masking. *Audiology*, 1971, **10**, 65-76.

Elman, J. L. Perceptual origins of the phoneme boundary effect and selective adaptation to speech: A signal detection analysis. *Journal of the Acoustical Society of America,*1979, **65**, 190-207.

Evans, C. R., & Wilson, J. Subjective changes in the perception of consonants when presented as "stabilized auditory images." *Division of Computer Science Publication No. 41, National Physical Laboratory* (England), November 1968.

Fant, C. G. M. Descriptive analysis of the acoustic aspects of speech. *Logos*, 1962, **5**, 3-17.

Fastl, H. Pulsation patterns of sinusoids vs. critical band noise. *Perception & Psychophysics*, 1975, **18**, 95-97.

Fay, W. H. *Temporal sequence in the perception of speech.* The Hague: Mouton, 1966.

Fechner, G. T. *Elemente der Psychophysik.* Leipzig: Breitkopf u. Härtel, 1860.

Feddersen, W. E., Sandel, T. T., Teas, D. C., & Jeffress, L. A. Localization of high-frequency tones. *Journal of the Acoustical Society of America*, 1957, **29**, 988-991.

Fettiplace, R., & Crawford, A. C. The origin of tuning in turtle cochlear hair cells. *Hearing Research*, 1980, **2**, 447-454.

Fieandt, K. von. Loudness invariance in sound perception. *Acta Psychologica Fennica*, 1951, **1**, 9-20.

Flanagan, J. L. *Speech analysis synthesis and perception.* (2nd Ed.) Berlin: Springer-Verlag, 1972.

Flanagan, J. L., & Guttman, N. On the pitch of periodic pulses.*Journal of the Acoustical Society of America*, 1960, **32**, 1308-1319. (a)

Flanagan, J. L., & Guttman, N. Pitch of periodic pulses without fundamental component. *Journal of the Acoustical Society of America*, 1960, **32**, 1319-1328. (b)

Fletcher, H. The physical criterion for determining the pitch of a musical tone. *Physical Review*, 1924, **23**, 427-437.

Fletcher, H. A space-time pattern theory of hearing. *Journal of the Acoustical Society of America*, 1930, **1**, 311-343.

Fletcher, H. Auditory patterns. *Review of Modern Physics*, 1940, **12**, 47-65.

Fletcher, H. *Speech and hearing in communication.* New York: Van Nostrand, 1953.

Flock, Å., Flock, B., & Murray, E. Studies on the sensory hairs of receptor cells in the inner ear. *Acta Otolaryngologica* (Stockholm), 1977, **83**, 85-91.

Foulke, E., & Sticht, T. G. Review of research on the intelligibility and comprehension of accelerated speech. *Psychological Bulletin,*1969, **72**, 50-62.

Fourcin, A. J. The pitch of noise with periodic spectral peaks. *Reports of the 5th International Congress on Acoustics* (Liège), 1965, 1A, B42.

Fourcin, A. J. Central pitch and auditory lateralization. In R. Plomp and G. F. Smoorenburg (Eds.), *Frequency analysis and periodicity detection in hearing.* Leiden, The Netherlands: Sijthoff, 1970, 319-328.

Fraisse, P. *The psychology of time* (J. Leith, Trans.). New York: Harper & Row, 1963.

Freedman, S. J., & Fisher, H. G. The role of the pinna in auditory localization. In S. J. Freedman (Ed.), *Neuropsychology of spatially oriented behavior.* Homewood, Ill.: Dorsey Press, 1968, 135-152.

Fromkin, V. A. The non-anomalous nature of anomalous utterances. *Language*, 1971, **47**, 27-52.

Fromkin, V. A. *Speech errors as linguistic evidence.* The Hague: Mouton, 1973.

Fromkin, V. A. Introduction. In V. A. Fromkin (Ed.), *Errors in linguistic performance: Slips of the tongue, ear, pen, and hand.* New York: Academic Press, 1980, 1-12.

Gacek, R. R. The efferent cochlear bundle in man. *Archives of Otolaryngology,* 1961, **74,** 690-694.

Gacek, R. R. Neuroanatomy of the auditory system. In J. V. Tobias (Ed.), *Foundations of modern auditory theory,* Vol. 2. New York: Academic Press, 1972, 241-262.

Gamble, E. A. McC. Minor studies from the psychological laboratory of Wellesley College, I. Intensity as a criterion in estimating the distance of sounds. *Psychological Review,* 1909, **16,** 416-426.

Gardner, M. B. Historical background of the Haas and/or precedence effect. *Journal of the Acoustical Society of America,* 1968, **43,** 1243-1248.

Gardner, M. B. Distance estimation of 0° or apparent 0°-oriented speech signals in anechoic space. *Journal of the Acoustical Society of America,* 1969, **45,** 47-53.

Gardner, M. B., & Gardner, R. S. Problem of localization in the median plane: Effect of pinnae cavity occlusion. *Journal of the Acoustical Society of America,* 1973, **53,** 400-408.

Garner, W. R. The accuracy of counting repeated short tones. *Journal of Experimental Psychology,* 1951, **41,** 310-316.

Garner, W. R. Context effects and the validity of loudness scales. *Journal of Experimental Psychology,* 1954, **48,** 218-224.

Garner, W. R., & Gottwald, R. L. Some perceptual factors in the learning of sequential patterns of binary events. *Journal of Verbal Learning and Verbal Behavior,* 1967, **6,** 582-589.

Garner, W. R., & Gottwald, R. L. The perception and learning of temporal patterns. *Quarterly Journal of Experimental Psychology,* 1968, **20,** 97-109.

Garnes, S., & Bond, Z. S. A slip of the ear: A snip of the ear? A slip of the year? In V. A. Fromkin (Ed.), *Errors in linguistic performance: Slips of the tongue, ear, pen, and hand.* New York: Academic Press, 1980, 231-239.

Gibson, E. J., & Levin, H. *The psychology of reading.* Cambridge, Mass.: MIT Press, 1975.

Gibson, J. J. Adaptation with negative after-effect. *Psychological Review,* 1937, **44,** 222-244.

Gibson, J. J. *The senses considered as perceptual systems.* Boston: Houghton Mifflin, 1966.

Gleitman, L. R., & Rozin, P. Teaching reading by use of a syllabary. *Reading Research Quarterly,* 1973, **8,** 447-483.

Gleitman, L. R., & Rozin, P. The structure and acquisition of reading, I: Relations between orthographies and the structure of language. In A. S. Reber and D. L. Scarborough (Eds.), *Toward a psychology of reading.* Hillsdale, N.J.: Erlbaum, 1977, 1-53.

Goldstein, J. L. An optimum processor theory for the central formation of the pitch of complex tones. *Journal of the Acoustical Society of America,* 1973, **54,** 1496-1516.

Goldstein, J. L. Mechanisms of signal analysis and pattern perception in periodicity pitch. *Audiology,* 1978, **17,** 421-445.

Goldstein, L. M., & Lackner, J. R. Alterations in the phonetic coding of speech sounds during repetition. *Cognition*, 1974, **2**, 279-297.

Gonshor, A., & Jones, G. M. Changes of human vestibulo-ocular response induced by vision-reversal during head rotation. *Journal of Physiology* (London), 1973, **234**, 102-103P.

Gray, G. W. Phonemic microtomy: The minimum duration of perceptible speech sounds. *Speech Monographs*, 1942, **9**, 75-90.

Graybiel, A., Kerr, W. A., & Bartley, S. H. Stimulus thresholds of the semicircular canals as a function of angular acceleration. *American Journal of Psychology*, 1948, **61**, 21-36.

Green, D. M. *An introduction to hearing.* Hillsdale, N.J.: Erlbaum, 1976.

Green, D. M., & Yost, W. A. Binaural analysis. In W. D. Keidel and W. D. Neff (Eds.), *Handbook of sensory physiology*, Vol. 2. Berlin: Springer-Verlag, 1975, 461-480.

Greenwood, D. D. Critical bandwidth and the frequency coordinates of the basilar membrane. *Journal of the Acoustical Society of America*, 1961, **33**, 1344-1356.

Guttman, N., & Flanagan, J. L. Pitch of high-pass filtered pulse trains. *Journal of the Acoustical Society of America*, 1964, **36**, 757-765.

Guttman, N., & Julesz, B. Lower limit of auditory periodicity analysis. *Journal of the Acoustical Society of America*, 1963, **35**, 610.

Hafter, E. R., & Carrier, S. C. Binaural interaction in low-frequency stimuli: The inability to trade time and intensity completely. *Journal of the Acoustical Society of America*, 1972, **51**, 1852-1862.

Hafter, E. R., Dye, R. H., Jr., & Gilkey, R. H. Lateralization of tonal signals which have neither onsets nor offsets. *Journal of the Acoustical Society of America*, 1979, **65**, 471-477.

Hafter, E. R., & Jeffress, L. A. Two-image lateralization of tones and clicks. *Journal of the Acoustical Society of America*, 1968, **44**, 563-569.

Halle, M., & Stevens, K. N. Speech recognition: A model and a program for research. In J. A. Fodor and J. J. Katz (Eds.), *The structure of language.* Englewood Cliffs, N.J.: Prentice-Hall, 1972, 604-612.

Ham, L. B., & Parkinson, J. S. Loudness and intensity relations. *Journal of the Acoustical Society of America*, 1932, **3**, 511-534.

Harris, G. G. Binaural interactions of impulsive stimuli and pure tones. *Journal of the Acoustical Society of America*, 1960, **32**, 685-692.

Heise, G. A., & Miller, G. A. An experimental study of auditory patterns. *American Journal of Psychology*, 1951, **64**, 68-77.

Held, R. Shifts in binaural localization after prolonged exposures to atypical combinations of stimuli. *American Journal of Psychology*, 1955, **68**, 526-548.

Helmholtz, H. L. F. *On the sensations of tone as a physiological basis for the theory of music.* New York: Dover, 1954. Reprint of 2nd English Edition of 1885 (A. J. Ellis, Trans.), based upon the 3rd German Edition (1870) and rendered conformal with the 4th German Edition (1877).

Helson, H. *Adaptation level theory: An experimental and systematic approach to behavior.* New York: Harper & Row, 1964.

Henning, G. B. Detectability of interaural delay in high-frequency complex waveforms. *Journal of the Acoustical Society of America*, 1974, **55**, 84-90.

Hirano, M., Ohala, J., & Vennard, W. The function of laryngeal muscles in regulating fundamental frequency and intensity of phonation. *Journal of Speech and Hearing Research*, 1969, **12**, 616-628.

Hirsh, I. J. The influence of interaural phase on interaural summation and inhibition. *Journal of the Acoustical Society of America*, 1948, **20**, 536-544. (a)

Hirsh, I. J. Binaural summation and interaural inhibition as a function of the level of the masking noise. *American Journal of Psychology*, 1948, **61**, 205-213. (b)

Hirsh, I. J. Auditory perception of temporal order. *Journal of the Acoustical Society of America*, 1959, **31**, 759-767.

Hirsh, I. J., & Sherrick, C. E. Perceived order in different sense modalities. *Journal of Experimental Psychology*, 1961, **62**, 423-432.

Holloway, C. M. Passing the strongly voiced components of noisy speech. *Nature*, 1970, **226**, 178-179.

Hood, D. C., & Finkelstein, M. A. On relating physiology to perception. *Behavioral and Brain Sciences*, 1981, **4**, 195.

Houtgast, T. Psychophysical evidence for lateral inhibition in hearing. *Journal of the Acoustical Society of America*, 1972, **51**, 1885-1894.

Houtgast, T. Psychophysical experiments on "tuning curves" and "two-tone inhibition." *Acustica*, 1973, **29**, 168-179.

Houtgast, T. *Lateral suppression in hearing*. Doctoral dissertation, Free University, Amsterdam, 1974. (a)

Houtgast, T. Masking patterns and lateral inhibition. In E. Zwicker and E. Terhardt (Eds.), *Facts and models in hearing*. Berlin: Springer-Verlag, 1974, 258-265. (b)

Houtgast, T. The slopes of the masking pattern. In E. Zwicker and E. Terhardt (Eds.), *Facts and models in hearing*. Berlin: Springer-Verlag, 1974, 269-272. (c)

Houtsma, A. J. M., & Goldstein, J. L. The central origin of the pitch of complex tones: Evidence from musical interval recognition. *Journal of the Acoustical Society of America*, 1972, **51**, 520-529.

Hudspeth, A. J., & Jacobs, R. Stereocilia mediate transduction in vertebrate hair cells. *Proceedings of the National Academy of Sciences* (U.S.A.), 1979, **76**, 1506-1509.

Huey, E. B. *The psychology and pedagogy of reading*. Cambridge, Mass.: MIT Press, 1968.

Huggins, A. W. F. Distortion of the temporal pattern of speech: Interruption and alternation. *Journal of the Acoustical Society of America*, 1964, **36**, 1055-1064.

Huizing, E. H., & Spoor, A. An unusual type of tinnitus. *Archives of Otolaryngology*, 1973, **98**, 134-136.

Hunt, H. V. *Origins in acoustics: The science of sound from antiquity to the age of Newton*. New Haven, Conn.: Yale University Press, 1978.

Jakobson, R., Fant, C. G. M., & Halle, M. *Preliminaries to speech analysis: The distinctive features and their correlates*. Cambridge, Mass.: MIT Press, 1963.

Johnstone, B. M., & Boyle, A. J. F. Basilar membrane vibration examined with the Mössbauer technique. *Science*, 1967, **158**, 389-390.

Johnstone, B. M., Taylor, K. J., & Boyle, A. J. Mechanics of the guinea pig cochlea. *Journal of the Acoustical Society of America*, 1970, **47**, 504-509.

Jongkees, L. B. W., & Veer, R. A. v. d. Directional hearing capacity in hearing disorders. *Acta Oto-Laryngologica*, 1957, **48**, 465-474.

Joos, M. Acoustic phonetics. Supplement to *Language*, 1948, **24**, 1-136 (*Language Monograph* No. 23).

Jusczyk, P. W., Smith, L. B., & Murphy, C. The perceptual classification of speech. *Perception & Psychophysics*, 1981, **30**, 10-23.

Kiang, N. Y.-S. *Discharge patterns of single fibers in the cat's auditory nerve.* (Research Monograph No. 35) Cambridge, Mass.: MIT Press, 1965.

Kimura, D. Functional asymmetry of the brain in dichotic listening. *Cortex*, 1967, **3**, 163-178.

Kinney, J. A. S. Discrimination of auditory and visual patterns. *American Journal of Psychology*, 1961, **74**, 529-541.

Kinsbourne, M. The cerebral basis of lateral asymmetries in attention. In A. F. Sanders (Ed.), *Attention and performance III.* Amsterdam: North Holland, 1970, 193-201.

Klatt, D. H. Speech perception: A model of acoustic-phonetic analysis and lexical access. *Journal of Phonetics*, 1979, **7**, 279-312.

Klumpp, R. G., & Eady, H. R. Some measurements of interaural time-difference thresholds. *Journal of the Acoustical Society of America*, 1956, **28**, 859-860.

Kock, W. E. Binaural localization and masking. *Journal of the Acoustical Society of America*, 1950, **22**, 801-804.

Kohllöffel, L. U. E. A study of basilar membrane vibrations. I. Fuzziness detection: A new method for the analysis of microvibrations with laser light. *Acustica*, 1972, **27**, 49-65. (a)

Kohllöffel, L. U. E. A study of basilar membrane vibrations. II. The vibratory amplitude and phase pattern along the basilar membrane (post mortem). *Acustica*, 1972, **27**, 66-81. (b)

Kohllöffel, L. U. E. A study of basilar membrane vibrations. III. The basilar membrane frequency response curve in the living guinea pig. *Acustica*, 1972, **27**, 82-89. (c)

Kries, J. von. Commentary. In J.P.C. Southall (Ed.), *Helmholtz's treatise on physiological optics,* Vol. 3. New York: Dover, 1962, 239. (Translated from the 3rd German Edition originally published in 1910.)

Kronberg, H., Mellert, V., & Schreiner, C. Dichotic and monaural pulsation thresholds. *Proceedings of the 8th International Congress on Acoustics* (London), 1974, **1**, 143.

Kuhl, P., & Miller, J. D. Discrimination of speech sounds by the chinchilla: /t/ vs. /d/ in CV syllables. *Journal of the Acoustical Society of America*, 1974, **56**, S52 (Abstract).

Kuhl, P., & Miller, J. D. Speech perception by the chinchilla: Identification functions for synthetic VOT stimuli. *Journal of the Acoustical Society of America*, 1978, **63**, 905-917.

Kuhn, G. F. Model for the interaural time differences in the azimuthal plane. *Journal of the Acoustical Society of America*, 1977, **62**, 157-167.

Kunov, H., & Abel, S. Effects of rise/decay time on the lateralization of interaurally delayed 1-kHz tones. *Journal of the Acoustical Society of America*, 1981, **69**, 769-773.

Ladefoged, P. The perception of speech. In *National Physical Laboratory Symposium No. 10, Mechanisation of Thought Processes.* Her Majesty's Stationery Office, London, 1959, **1**, 309-417.

Ladefoged, P., & Broadbent, D. E. Perception of sequence in auditory events. *Quarterly Journal of Experimental Psychology*, 1960, **12**, 162-170.

Laird, D. A., Taylor, E., & Wille, H. H. The apparent reduction of loudness. *Journal of the Acoustical Society of America*, 1932, **3**, 393-401.

Lane, C. E. Binaural beats. *Physical Review*, 1925, **26**, 401-412.

Lane, H. L., Catania, A. C., & Stevens, S. S. Voice level: Autophonic scale, perceived loudness, and effects of sidetone. *Journal of the Acoustical Society of America*, 1961, **33**, 160-167.

Langmuir, I., Schaefer, V. J., Ferguson, C. V., & Hennelly, E. F. A study of binaural perception of the direction of a sound source. *OSRD Report No. 4079*, Publ. No. 31014 (June 30, 1944). (Available from the United States Department of Commerce.)

Lashley, K. S. The problem of serial order in behavior. In L. A. Jeffress (Ed.), *Cerebral mechanisms in behavior: The Hixon Symposium*. New York: Wiley, 1951, 112-136.

Lawrence, M. Middle ear muscle influence on binaural hearing. *Archives of Otolaryngology*, 1965, **82**, 478-482.

Lawrence, M., & Yantis, P. A. Onset and growth of aural harmonics in the overloaded ear. *Journal of the Acoustical Society of America*, 1956, **28**, 852-858.

Layton, B. Differential effects of two nonspeech sounds on phonemic restoration. *Bulletin of the Psychonomic Society*, 1975, **6**, 487-490.

Lazarus-Mainka, G., & Hörmann, H. Strategic selection (metacontrol) of hemisphere dominance in normal human subjects. *Psychological Research*, 1978, **40**, 15-25.

Leshowitz, B. Measurement of the auditory stimulus. In E. C. Carterette and M. P. Friedman (Eds.), *Handbook of perception*, Vol 4.New York: Academic Press, 1978, 83-124.

Levy, E. T., & Butler, R. A. Stimulus factors which influence the perceived externalization of sound presented through headphones. *Journal of Auditory Research*, 1978, **18**, 41-50.

Lewis, B., & Coles, R. Sound localization in birds. *Trends in NeuroSciences*, 1980, **3**, 102-105.

Liberman, A. M., Cooper, F. S., Shankweiler, D. P., & Studdert-Kennedy, M. Perception of the speech code. *Psychological Review*, 1967, **74**, 431-46l.

Liberman, A. M., Delattre, P., & Cooper, F. S. The role of selected stimulus-variables in the perception of the unvoiced stop consonants. *American Journal of Psychology*, 1952, **65**, 497-516.

Liberman, I. Y., Shankweiler, D., Fischer, F. W., & Carter, B. Reading and the awareness of linguistic segments. *Journal of Experimental Child Psychology*, 1974, **18**, 201-212.

Licklider, J. C. R. "Periodicity" pitch and "place" pitch. *Journal of the Acoustical Society of America*, 1954, **26**, 945 (Abstract).

Lieberman, P. Some effects of semantic and grammatical context on the production and perception of speech. *Language and Speech*, 1963, **6**, 172-187.

Lim, D. J. Cochlear anatomy related to cochlear micromechanics. A review. *Journal of the Acoustical Society of America*, 1980, **67**, 1686-1695.

Lindsay, P. H., & Norman, D. A. *Human information processing: An introduction to psychology*. (2nd Ed.) New York: Academic Press, 1977.

Lüdtke, H. Die Alphabetschrift und das Problem der Lautsegmentierung. *Phonetica,* 1969, **20,** 147-176.

MacNeilage, P. F. Motor control of serial ordering in speech. *Psychological Review,* 1970, **77,** 182-196.

MacNeilage, P., & Ladefoged, P. The production of speech and language. In E. C. Carterette and M. P. Friedman, *Handbook of perception,* Vol. 7. *Language and speech.* New York: Academic Press, 1976, 75-120.

Mansfield, R. J. W. Sensory coding: The search for invariants. *Behavioral and Brain Sciences,* 1981, **4,** 198-199.

Marks, L. E. *The unity of the senses: Interrelations among the modalities.* New York: Academic Press, 1978.

Massaro, D. W. Reading and listening (tutorial paper). In P. A. Kolers, M. E. Wrolstad, and H. Bouma (Eds.), *Processing of visible language.* New York: Plenum, 1979, 331-354.

Matsumoto, M. Researches on acoustic space. In E. W. Scripture (Ed.), *Studies from the Yale psychological laboratory,* 1897, **5,** 1-75.

Maxfield, J. P. Acoustic control of recording for talking motion pictures. *Journal of the Society of Motion Picture Engineers,* 1930, **14,** 85-95.

Maxfield, J. P. Some physical factors affecting the illusion in sound motion pictures. *Journal of the Acoustical Society of America,* 1931, **3,** 69-80.

McFadden, D., & Pasanen, E. G. Binaural beats at high frequencies. *Science,* 1975, **190,** 394-396.

McGurk, H., & MacDonald, J. Hearing lips and seeing voices. *Nature,* 1976, **264,** 746-748.

Meringer, R., & Mayer, C. *Versprechen und Verlesen: Eine psychologische-linguistische Studie.* Stuttgart: Göschensche Verlagsbuchhandlung, 1895.

Mershon, D. H., & Bowers, J. N. Absolute and relative cues for the auditory perception of egocentric distance. *Perception,* 1979, **8,** 311-322.

Mershon, D. H., & King, L. E. Intensity and reverberation as factors in the auditory perception of egocentric distance. *Perception & Psychophysics,* 1975, **18,** 409-415.

Meyer, M. F. Aural harmonics are fictitious. *Journal of the Acoustical Society of America,* 1957, **29,** 749.

Miller, G. A. Decision units in the perception of speech. *IRE Transactions on Information Theory,* 1962. **IT-8,** 81-83.

Miller, G. A., & Licklider, J. C. R. The intelligibility of interrupted speech. *Journal of the Acoustical Society of America,* 1950. **22,** 167-173.

Miller, R. L. Masking effects of periodically pulsed tones as a function of time and frequency. *Journal of the Acoustical Society of America,* 1947, **19,** 798-807.

Mills, A. W. On the minimum audible angle. *Journal of the Acoustical Society of America,* 1958, **30,** 237-246.

Mills, A. W. Auditory localization. In J. V. Tobias (Ed.), *Foundations of modern auditory theory,* Vol. 2. New York: Academic Press, 1972, 303-348.

Mohrmann, K. Lautheitskonstanz im Entfernungswechsel. *Zeitschrift für Psychologie,* 1939, **145,** 145-199.

Monroe, M. *Children who cannot read.* Chicago: University of Chicago Press, 1932.

Moore, B. C. J. Relation between the critical bandwidth and the frequency-difference limen. *Journal of the Acoustical Society of America,* 1974, **55,** 359.

Moore, B. C. J. *Introduction to the psychology of hearing.* Baltimore, Md.: University Park Press, 1977.

Moore, M. W., & Bliss, J. C. The Optacon reading system. *Education of the Visually Handicapped,* 1975, **7,** 15-21.

Moore, T. J., & Mundie, J. R. Specification of the minimum number of glottal pulses necessary for reliable identification of selected speech sounds. *Aerospace Medical Research Laboratory Report,* 1971, TR-70-104.

Morais, J., Cary, L., Alegria, J., & Bertelson, P. Does awareness of speech as a sequence of phones arise spontaneously? *Cognition,* 1979, **7,** 323-331.

Naeser, M. A., & Lilly, J. C. Preliminary evidence for a universal detector system— Perception of the repeating word. *Journal of the Acoustical Society of America,* 1970, **48,** 85 (Abstract).

Negus, V. E. *The comparative anatomy and physiology of the larynx.* New York: Grune & Stratton, 1949.

Neisser, U. *Cognitive psychology.* New York: Appleton, 1967.

Neisser, U., & Hirst, W. Effect of practice on the identification of auditory sequences. *Perception & Psychophysics,* 1974, **15,** 391-398.

Newton, I. *Opticks, or a treatise of the reflections, refractions, inflections & colours of light.* (4th Ed.) London, 1730. (Reprinted New York: Dover, 1952.)

Nickerson, R. S., & Freeman, B. Discrimination of the order of the components of repeating tone sequences: Effects of frequency separation and extensive practice. *Perception & Psychophysics,* 1974, **16,** 471-477.

Noorden, L.P.A.S., Van. *Temporal coherence in the perception of tone sequences.* Doctoral dissertation, Eindhoven University of Technology (The Netherlands), 1975.

Noorden, L.P.A.S., Van, Minimum differences of level and frequency for perceptual fission of tone sequences ABAB. *Journal of the Acoustical Society of America,* 1977, **61,** 1041-1045.

Nordmark, J. O. Mechanisms of frequency discrimination. *Journal of the Acoustical Society of America,* 1968, **44,** 1533-1540.

Norman, D. A. Temporal confusions and limited capacity processors. *Acta Psychologica,* 1967, **27,** 293-297.

Obusek, C. J., & Warren, R. M. Relation of the verbal transformation and the phonemic restoration effects. *Cognitive Psychology,* 1973, **5,** 97-107.

Ohm, G. S. Ueber die Definition des Tones, nebst daran geknüpfter Theorie der Sirene und ähnlicher tonbildender Vorrichtungen. *Annalen der Physik und Chemie,* 1843, **59,** 513-565.

Ohm, G. S. Noch ein Paar Worte über die Definition des Tones. *Annalen der Physik und Chemie,* 1844, **62,** 1-18.

Öhman, S. E. G. Perception of segments of VCCV utterances. *Journal of the Acoustical Society of America,* 1966, **40,** 979-988.

Opheim, O., & Flottorp, G. The aural harmonics in normal and pathological hearing. *Acta Oto-Laryngologica,* 1955, **45,** 513-531.

Ortmann, O. On the melodic relativity of tones. *Psychological Monographs*, 1926, **35** (1, Whole No. 162).

Paivio, A. *Imagery and verbal processes*. New York: Holt, Rinehart & Winston, 1971.

Paivio, A., & Csapo, K. Concrete-image and verbal memory codes. *Journal of Experimental Psychology*, 1969, **80**, 279-285.

Patterson, J. H., & Green, D. M. Discrimination of transient signals having identical energy spectra. *Journal of the Acoustical Society of America*, 1970, **48**, 894-905.

Patterson, R. D. Noise masking of a change in residue pitch. *Journal of the Acoustical Society of America*, 1969, **45**, 1520-1524.

Peake, W. T., & Ling, A., Jr. Basilar-membrane motion in the alligator lizard: Its relation to tonotopic organization and frequency selectivity. *Journal of the Acoustical Society of America*, 1980, **67**, 1736-1745.

Peterson, G. E. Influence of voice quality. *Volta Review*, 1946, **48**, 640-641.

Peterson, G. E., & Barney, H. L. Control methods used in a study of the vowels. *Journal of the Acoustical Society of America*, 1952, **24**, 115-184.

Philipchalk, R., & Rowe, F. J. Sequential and nonsequential memory for verbal and nonverbal auditory stimuli. *Journal of Experimental Psychology*, 1971, **91**, 341-343.

Pickett, J. M. *The sounds of speech communication: A primer of acoustic phonetics and speech perception*. Baltimore, Md.: University Park Press, 1980.

Pierce, A. H. *Studies in auditory and visual space perception*. New York: Longmans, Green, 1901.

Piston, W. *Counterpoint*. New York: Norton, 1947.

Plateau, J. Sur la mesure des sensations physiques, et sur la loi qui lie l'intensité de ces sensations à l'intensité de la cause excitante. *Bulletins de l'Académie Royale des Sciences, des Lettres et des Beaux-Arts de Belgique*, 1872, **33**, 376-388 (Série 2).

Plenge, G. On the differences between localization and lateralization. *Journal of the Acoustical Society of America*, 1974, **56**, 944-951.

Plomp, R. The ear as a frequency analyzer. *Journal of the Acoustical Society of America*, 1964, **36**, 1628-1636.

Plomp, R. *Experiments on tone perception*. Doctoral dissertation, University of Utrecht (The Netherlands), 1966.

Plomp, R. Beats of mistuned consonances. *Journal of the Acoustical Society of America*, 1967, **42**, 462-474.

Plomp, R. *Aspects of tone sensation*. London: Academic Press, 1976.

Plomp, R., & Levelt, W. J. M. Tonal consonance and critical bandwidth. *Journal of the Acoustical Society of America*, 1965, **38**, 548-560.

Plomp, R., & Mimpen, A. M. The ear as a frequency analyzer. II. *Journal of the Acoustical Society of America*, 1968, **43**, 764-767.

Polanyi, M. *Personal knowledge*. Chicago: Chicago University Press, 1958.

Polanyi, M. Logic and psychology. *American Psychologist*, 1968, **23**, 27-43.

Pollack, I. On the measurement of the loudness of speech. *Journal of the Acoustical Society of America*, 1952, **24**, 323-324.

Potter, R. K., Kopp, G. A., & Kopp, H. G. *Visible speech*. New York: Van Nostrand, 1947. (Reprinted New York: Dover, 1966.)

Poulton, E. C., & Freeman, P. R. Unwanted asymmetrical transfer effects with balanced experimental designs. *Psychological Bulletin*, 1966, **66**, 1-8.

Powers, G. L., & Wilcox, J. C. Intelligibility of temporally interrupted speech with and without intervening noise. *Journal of the Acoustical Society of America,* 1977, **61,** 195-199.

Preusser, D. The effect of structure and rate on the recognition and description of auditory temporal patterns. *Perception & Psychophysics,* 1972, **11,** 233-240.

Prohovnik, I. Cerebral lateralization of psychological processes: A literature review. *Archiv für Psychologie,* 1978, **130,** 161-211.

Rasmussen, G. L. The olivary peduncle and other fiber projections of the superior olivary complex. *Journal of Comparative Neurology,* 1946, **84,** 141-219.

Rasmussen, G. L. Further observations of the efferent cochlear bundle. *Journal of Comparative Neurology,* 1953, **99,** 61-74.

Rayleigh, Lord. On our perception of sound direction. *Philosophical Magazine,* 1907, **13,** 214-232.

Reisz, R. R. Differential sensitivity of the ear for pure tones. *Physical Review,* 1928, **31,** 867-875.

Remez, R. E. Adaptation of the category boundary between speech and non-speech: A case against feature detectors. *Cognitive Psychology,* 1979, **11,** 38-57.

Rhode, W. S. Observations of the vibration of the basilar membrane in squirrel monkeys using the Mössbauer technique. *Journal of the Acoustical Society of America,* 1971, **49,** 1218-1231.

Rhode, W. S. An investigation of post-mortem cochlear mechanics using the Mössbauer effect. In A. R. Møller (Ed.), *Basic mechanisms in hearing.* New York: Academic Press, 1973, 49-67.

Richardson, L. F., & Ross, J. S. Loudness and telephone current. *Journal of General Psychology,* 1930, **3,** 288-306.

Riesen, A. H. (Ed.) *The developmental neuropsychology of sensory deprivation.* New York: Academic Press, 1975.

Ritsma, R. J. Existence region of the tonal residue. I. *Journal of the Acoustical Society of America,* 1962, **34,** 1224-1229.

Ritsma, R. J. Existence region of the tonal residue. II. *Journal of the Acoustical Society of America,* 1963, **35,** 1241-1245.

Ritsma, R. J. Periodicity detection. In R. Plomp and G. F. Smoorenburg (Eds.), *Frequency analysis and periodicity detection in hearing.* Leiden, The Netherlands: Sijthoff, 1970, 250-266.

Roffler, S. K., & Butler, R. A. Factors that influence the localization of sound in the vertical plane. *Journal of the Acoustical Society of America,* 1968, **43,** 1255-1259.

Rose, J. E., Brugge, J. F., Anderson, D. J., & Hind, J. E. Phase-locked response to low-frequency tones in single auditory nerve fibers of the squirrel monkey. *Journal of Neurophysiology,* 1967, **30,** 769-793.

Rose, J. E., Hind, J. E., Anderson, D. J., & Brugge, J. F. Some effects of stimulus intensity on response of auditory nerve fibers in the squirrel monkey. *Journal of Neurophysiology,* 1971, **34,** 685-699.

Rosen, S. M. Range and frequency effects in consonant categorization. *Journal of Phonetics,* 1979, **7,** 393-402.

Rosen, S. M., Fourcin, A. J., & Moore, B. C. J. Voice pitch as an aid to lipreading. *Nature,* 1981, **291,** 150-152.

Roth, G. L., Kochhar, R. K., & Hind, J. E. Interaural time differences: Implications regarding the neurophysiology of sound localization. *Journal of the Acoustical Society of America*, 1980, **68**, 1643-1651.

Rowe, E. J., & Cake, L. J. Retention of order information for sounds and words. *Canadian Journal of Psychology*, 1977, **31**, 14-23.

Rowley, R. R., & Studebaker, G. A. Monaural loudness-intensity relationships for a 1,000-Hz tone. *Journal of the Acoustical Society of America*, 1969, **45**, 1186-1192.

Royer, F. L., & Garner, W. R. Perceptual organization of nine-element auditory temporal patterns. *Perception & Psychophysics*, 1970, **7**, 115-120.

Rozin, P., Poritsky, S., & Sotsky, R. American children with reading problems can easily learn to read English represented by Chinese characters. *Science*, 1971, **171**, 1264-1267.

Sachs, C. *Rhythm and tempo*. New York: Norton, 1953.

Samuel, A. G. The role of bottom-up confirmation in the phonemic restoration illusion. *Journal of Experimental Psychology: Human Perception and Performance*, 1981, **7**, 1124-1131. (a)

Samuel, A. G. Phonemic restoration: Insights from a new methodology. *Journal of Experimental Psychology: General*, 1981, **110**, 474-494. (b)

Sandel, T. T., Teas, D. C., Feddersen, W. E., & Jeffress, L.A. Localization of sound from single and paired sources. *Journal of the Acoustical Society of America*, 1955, **27**, 842-852.

Sasaki, T. Sound restoration and temporal localization of noise in speech and music sounds. *Tohuku Psychologica Folia*, 1980, **39**, 79-88.

Savin, H. B. What the child knows about speech when he starts to learn to read. In J. F. Kavanagh and I. G. Mattingly (Eds.), *Language by ear and by eye*. Cambridge, Mass.: MIT Press, 1972, 319-329.

Savin, H. B., & Bever, T. G. The nonperceptual reality of the phoneme. *Journal of Verbal Learning and Verbal Behavior*, 1970, **9**, 295-302.

Sawusch, J. R., & Nusbaum, H. C. Contextual effects in vowel perception. I: Anchor-induced contrast effects. *Perception & Psychophysics*, 1979, **25**, 292-302.

Scharf, B. Critical bands. In J. V. Tobias (Ed.), *Foundations of modern auditory theory*. Vol. 1. New York: Academic Press, 1970, 157-202.

Schouten, J. F. The perception of subjective tones. *K. Akademie van Wetenschappen, Amsterdam. Afdeeling Natuurkunde* (Proceedings), 1938, **41**, 1086-1093.

Schouten, J. F. Synthetic sound. *Philips Technical Review*, 1939, **4**, 153-180.

Schouten, J. F. The residue, a new component in subjective sound analysis. *K. Akademie van Wetenschappen, Amsterdam. Afdeeling Natuurkunde* (Proceedings), 1940, **43**, 356-365. (a)

Schouten, J. F. The perception of pitch. *Philips Technical Review*, 1940, **5**, 286-294. (b)

Schouten, J. F. The residue and the mechanism of hearing. *K. Akademie van Wetenschappen, Amsterdam. Afdeeling Natuurkunde* (Proceedings), 1940, **43**, 991-999. (c)

Schouten, J. F. The residue revisited. In R. Plomp and G .F. Smoorenburg (Eds.), *Frequency analysis and periodicity detection in hearing*. Leiden, The Netherlands: Sijthoff, 1970, 41-58.

Schouten, J. F., Ritsma, R. J., & Cardozo, B. L. Pitch of the residue. *Journal of the Acoustical Society of America*, 1962, **34**, 1418-1424.

Schreiner, C., Gottlob, D., & Mellert, V. Influences of the pulsation threshold method on psychoacoustical tuning curves. *Acustica*, 1977, **37**, 29-36.

Schultz, D. P. *Sensory restriction: Effects on behavior*. New York: Academic Press, 1965.

Searle, C. L., Jacobson, J. Z., & Rayment, S. G. Stop consonant discrimination based on human audition. *Journal of the Acoustical Society of America*, 1979, **65**, 799-809.

Seebeck, A. Beobachtungen über einige Bedingungen der Enstehung von Tönen. *Annalen der Physik und Chemie*, 1841, **53**, 417-437.

Seebeck, A. Ueber die Sirene. *Annalen der Physik und Chemie*, 1843, **60**, 449-481.

Seebeck, A. Ueber die Definition des Tones. *Annalen der Physik und Chemie*, 1844, **63**, 353-368.

Severance, E. & Washburn, M. F. Minor studies from the psychological laboratory of Vassar College. IV. The loss of associative power in words after long fixation. *American Journal of Psychology*, 1907, **18**, 182-186.

Shankweiler, D., & Liberman, I. Y. Misreading: A search for causes. In J. F. Kavanagh and I. G. Mattingly (Eds.), *Language by ear and by eye*. Cambridge, Mass.: MIT Press, 1972, 293-317.

Shattuck, S. R. *Speech errors and sentence production*. Doctoral dissertation, Massachusetts Institute of Technology, 1975.

Shaxby, J. H., & Gage, F. H. Studies in the localisation of sound. *Medical Research Council Special Report*, 1932, Series No. *166*, 1-32.

Sherman, G. L. *The phonemic restoration effect: An insight into the mechanisms of speech perception*. Unpublished M. S. dissertation, University of Wisconsin-Milwaukee, 1971.

Shigenaga, S. The constancy of loudness and of acoustic distance. In Y. Akishige (Ed.), *Bulletin of the Faculty of Literature. Kyushu University*, 1965, **9**, 289-333.

Shutt, C. E. Experiments in judging the distance of sound. *Kansas University Quarterly*, 1898, **7A**, 1-8.

Silverman, S. R., & Hirsh, I. J. Problems related to the use of speech in clinical audiometry. *Annals of Otology, Rhinology, and Laryngology*, 1955, **64**, 1234-1245.

Simmons, F. B. Perceptual theories of middle ear function. *Annals of Otology, Rhinology, and Laryngology*, 1964, **73**, 724-740.

Simon, H. J. & Studdert-Kennedy, M. Selective anchoring and adaptation of phonetic and nonphonetic continua. *Journal of the Acoustical Society of America*, 1978, **64**, 1338-1357.

Sinnott, J. M., Beecher, M.D., Moody, D. B., & Stebbins, W. C. Speech sound discrimination by monkeys and humans. *Journal of the Acoustical Society of America*, 1976, **60**, 687-695.

Skinner, B. F. The verbal summator and a method for the study of latent speech. *Journal of Psychology*, 1936, **2**, 71-107.

Small, A. M., Jr., & Campbell, R. A. Masking of pulsed tones by bands of noise. *Journal of the Acoustical Society of America*, 1961, **33**, 1570-1576.

Sperling, G., & Reeves, G. Measuring the reaction time of a shift of visual attention. In R. S. Nickerson (Ed.), *Attention and performance VIII*. Hillsdale, N.J.: Erlbaum, 1980, 347-360.

Spiegel, M. F. Thresholds for tones in maskers of various bandwidths as a function of signal frequency. *Journal of the Acoustical Society of America*, 1981, **69**, 791-795.

Starch, D., & Crawford, A. L. The perception of the distance of sound. *Psychological Review*, 1909, **16**, 427-430.

Steinberg, J. C., & Snow, W. B. Physical factors. *Bell System Technical Journal*, 1934, **13**, 245-258.

Stevens, K. N. Toward a model of speech recognition. *Journal of the Acoustical Society of America*, 1960, **32**, 47-55.

Stevens, K. N. The role of rapid spectrum changes in the production and perception of speech. In L. L. Hammerlich and R. Jakobson (Eds.), *Form and substance: Festschrift for Eli Fischer-Jørgensen*. Copenhagen: Akademisk Forlag, 1971, 95-101.

Stevens, K. N., & Blumstein, S. E. The search for invariant acoustic correlates of phonetic features. In P. D. Eimas and J. L. Miller (Eds.), *Perspectives on the study of speech*. Hillsdale, N.J.: Erlbaum, 1981, 1-38.

Stevens, K. N., & Halle, M. Remarks on analysis by synthesis and distinctive features. In W. Wathen-Dunn (Ed.), *Models for the perception of speech and visual form*. Cambridge, Mass.: MIT Press, 1967, 88-102.

Stevens, S. S. The measurement of loudness. *Journal of the Acoustical Society of America*, 1955, **27**, 815-829.

Stevens, S. S. The psychophysics of sensory function. In W. A. Rosenblith (Ed.), *Sensory communication*. New York: Wiley, 1961.

Stevens, S. S. Perceived level of noise by Mark VII and decibels (E). *Journal of the Acoustical Society of America*, 1972, **51**, 575-601.

Stevens, S. S. *Psychophysics: Introduction to its perceptual, neural and social prospects*. G. Stevens (Ed.). New York: Wiley, 1975.

Stevens, S. S., & Guirao, M. Loudness, reciprocality and partition scales. *Journal of the Acoustical Society of America*, 1962, **34**, 1466-1471.

Stevens, S. S., & Newman, E. B. The localization of actual sources of sound. *American Journal of Psychology*, 1936, **48**, 297-306.

Stevens, S. S., Volkmann, J., & Newman, E. B. A scale for the measurement of the psychological magnitude pitch. *Journal of the Acoustical Society of America*, 1937, **8**, 185-190.

Stuhlman, O., Jr. *An introduction to biophysics*. New York: Wiley, 1943.

Supa, M., Cotzin, M., & Dallenbach, K. M. "Facial vision": The perception of obstacles by the blind. *American Journal of Psychology*, 1944, **57**, 133-183.

Tallal, P., & Piercy, M. Defects of non-verbal auditory perception in children with developmental aphasia. *Nature*, 1973, **241**, 468-469.

Tallal, P., & Piercy, M. Developmental aphasia: Rate of auditory processing and selective impairment of consonant perception. *Neuropsychologia*, 1974, **12**, 83-93.

Talley, C. H. A comparison of conversational and audience speech. *Archives of Speech*, 1937, **2**, 28-40.

Teranishi, R. Critical rate for identification and information capacity in hearing system. *Journal of the Acoustical Society of Japan*, 1977, **33**, 136-143.

Terhardt, E. Pitch, consonance, and harmony. *Journal of the Acoustical Society of America*, 1974, **55**, 1061-1069.

Thomas, I. B., Cetti, R. P., & Chase, P. W. Effect of silent intervals on the perception of temporal order for vowels. *Journal of the Acoustical Society of America*, 1971, **49**, 84 (Abstract).

Thomas, I. B., & Fitzgibbons, P. J. Temporal order and perceptual classes. *Journal of the Acoustical Society of America*, 1971, **50**, 86-87 (Abstract).

Thomas, I. B., Hill, P. B., Carroll, F. S., & Garcia, B. Temporal order in the perception of vowels. *Journal of the Acoustical Society of America*, 1970, **48**, 1010-1013.

Thompson, R. K. R. *Performance of the bottlenose dolphin (Tursiops truncatus) on delayed auditory sequences and delayed auditory successive discriminations.* Doctoral dissertation, University of Hawaii, 1976.

Thompson, S. P. On the function of two ears in the perception of space. *The London, Edinburgh, and Dublin Philosophical Magazine and Journal of Science*, Series 5, 1882, **13**, 406-416.

Thurlow, W. R. An auditory figure-ground effect. *American Journal of Psychology*, 1957, **70**, 653-654.

Thurlow, W. R. Perception of low auditory pitch: A multicue, mediation theory. *Psychological Review*, 1963, **70**, 461-470.

Thurlow, W. R., & Elfner, L. F. Continuity effects with alternately sounding tones. *Journal of the Acoustical Society of America*, 1959, **31**, 1337-1339.

Thurlow, W. R., & Erchul, W. P. Understanding continuity effects with complex stimuli. *Journal of the American Auditory Society*, 1978, **4**, 113-116.

Thurlow, W. R., & Marten, A. E. Perception of steady and intermittent sound with alternating noise-burst stimuli. *Journal of the Acoustical Society of America*, 1962, **34**, 1853-1858.

Titchener, E. B. *A beginner's psychology.* New York: Macmillan, 1915.

Tobias, J. V., & Schubert, E. D. Effective onset duration of auditory stimuli. *Journal of the Acoustical Society of America*, 1959, **31**, 1595-1605.

Tonndorf, J. Shearing motion in scala media of cochlear models. *Journal of the Acoustical Society of America*, 1960, **32**, 238-244.

Tonndorf, J. Cochlear mechanics and hydro-dynamics. In J. V. Tobias (Ed.), *Foundations of modern auditory theory*, Vol. 1. New York: Academic Press, 1970, 203-254.

Tonndorf, J., & Khanna, S. M. Tympanic-membrane vibrations in human cadaver ears studied by time-averaged holography. *Journal of the Acoustical Society of America*, 1972, **52**, 1221-1233.

Tumarkin, A. A biologist looks at psycho-acoustics. *Journal of Sound and Vibration*, 1972, **21**, 115-126.

Vernon, J. *Inside the black room.* New York: Potter, 1963.

Verschuure, J. Transient phenomena in pulsation threshold measurement. *Audiology*, 1974, **13**, 90.

Verschuure, J. Pulsation threshold patterns and neuro-physiological tuning. In E. F. Evans and J. P. Wilson (Eds.), *Psychophysics and physiology of hearing*. London: Academic Press, 1977, 237-247.

Verschuure, J. *Auditory excitation patterns: The significance of the pulsation threshold method for the measurement of auditory nonlinearity.* Doctoral dissertation, Erasmus University (Rotterdam), 1978.

Verschuure, J., Rodenburg, M., & Maas, A. J. J. Frequency selectivity and temporal effects of the pulsation threshold method. *Proceedings of the 8th International Congress on Acoustics* (London), 1974, **1**, 131.

Vicario, G. L'*effetto tunnel acustico*. *Rivista di Psicologia*, 1960, **54**, 41-52.

Voldrich, L. Mechanical properties of basilar membrane. *Acta Otolaryngology*, 1978, **86**, 331-335.

Ward, W. D. Subjective musical pitch. *Journal of the Acoustical Society of America*, 1954, **26**, 369-380.

Warfield, D., Ruben, R. J., & Glackin, R. Word discrimination in cats. *Journal of Auditory Research*, 1966, **6**, 97-119.

Warren, R. M. A basis for judgments of sensory intensity. *American Journal of Psychology*, 1958, **71**, 675-687.

Warren, R. M. Illusory changes of distinct speech upon repetition—The verbal transformation effect. *British Journal of Psychology*, 1961, **52**, 249-258. (a)

Warren, R. M. Illusory changes in repeated words: Differences between young adults and the aged. *American Journal of Psychology*, 1961, **74**, 506-516. (b)

Warren, R. M. Are 'autophonic' judgments based on loudness? *American Journal of Psychology*, 1962, **75**, 452-456.

Warren, R. M. Vocal compensation for change in distance. *Proceedings of the 6th International Congress of Acoustics* (Tokyo), 1968, **A**, 61-64. (a)

Warren, R. M. Relation of verbal transformations to other perceptual phenomena. Conference Publication No. 42, *Institution of Electrical Engineers* (London), 1968, Supplement No. 1, 1-8. (b)

Warren, R. M. Verbal transformation effect and auditory perceptual mechanisms. *Psychological Bulletin*, 1968, **70**, 261-270. (c)

Warren, R. M. Elimination of biases in loudness judgments for tones. *Journal of the Acoustical Society of America*, 1970, **48**, 1397-1403. (a)

Warren, R. M. Perceptual restoration of missing speech sounds. *Science*, 1970, **167**, 392-393. (b)

Warren, R. M. Identification times for phonemic components of graded complexity and for spelling of speech. *Perception & Psychophysics*, 1971, **9**, 358-363.

Warren, R. M. Perception of temporal order: Special rules for initial and terminal sounds of sequences. *Journal of the Acoustical Society of America*, 1972, **52**, 167 (Abstract).

Warren, R. M. Quantification of loudness. *American Journal of Psychology*, 1973, **86**, 807-825. (b)

Warren, R. M. Anomalous loudness function of speech. *Journal of the Acoustical Society of America*, 1973, **54**, 390-396. (b)

Warren, R. M. Auditory temporal discrimination by trained listeners. *Cognitive Psychology*, 1974, **6**, 237-256. (a)

Warren, R. M. Auditory pattern discrimination by untrained listeners. *Perception & Psychophysics*, 1974, **15**, 495-500. (b)

Warren, R. M. Auditory illusions and perceptual processes. In N.J. Lass (Ed.), *Contemporary issues in experimental phonetics*. New York: Academic Press, 1976, 389-417. (a)

Warren, R. M. Auditory perception and speech evolution. In S. R. Harnad, H.D. Steklis, and J. Lancaster (Eds.), *Origins and evolution of language and speech*. New York: New York Academy of Sciences, 1976, 708-717. (b)

Warren, R.M. Subjective loudness and its physical correlate. *Acustica*, 1977, **37**, 334-346. (a)

Warren, R. M. Les illusions verbales. *La Recherche*, 1977, **8**, 538-543. (b)

Warren, R. M. Complex beats. *Journal of the Acoustical Society of America*, 1978, **64**, S38 (Abstract).

Warren, R. M. Measurement of sensory intensity. *Behavioral and Brain Sciences*, 1981, **4**, 175-189 (Target Article); 213-223 (Response to Open Peer Commentaries). (a)

Warren, R. M. Perceptual transformations in vision and hearing. *International Journal of Man-Machine Studies*, 1981, **14**, 123-132. (b)

Warren, R. M., & Ackroff, J. M. Two types of auditory sequence perception. *Perception & Psychophysics*, 1976, **20**, 387-394. (a)

Warren, R. M., & Ackroff, J. M. Dichotic verbal transformations and evidence of separate processors for identical stimuli. *Nature*, 1976, **259**, 475-477. (b)

Warren, R. M., & Bashford, J.A. Auditory contralateral induction: An early stage in binaural processing. *Perception & Psychophysics*, 1976, **20**, 380-386.

Warren, R. M., & Bashford, J. A., Jr. Perception of acoustic iterance: Pitch and infrapitch. *Perception & Psychophysics*, 1981, **29**, 395-402.

Warren, R. M., Bashford, J.A., Jr., & Wrightson, J. M. Infrapitch echo. *Journal of the Acoustical Society of America*, 1980, **68**, 1301-1305.

Warren, R. M., Bashford, J.A., Jr., & Wrightson, J. M. Detection of long interaural delays for broadband noise. *Journal of the Acoustical Society of America*, 1981, **69**, 1510-1514.

Warren, R. M., & Byrnes, D. L. Temporal discrimination of recycled tonal sequences: Pattern matching and naming of order by untrained listeners. *Perception & Psychophysics*, 1975, **18**, 273-280.

Warren, R. M., & Gregory, R. L. An auditory analogue of the visual reversible figure. *American Journal of Psychology*, 1958, **71**, 612-613.

Warren, R. M., & Obusek, C. J. Speech perception and phonemic restorations. *Perception & Psychophysics*, 1971, **9**, 358-362.

Warren, R. M., & Obusek, C. J. Identification of temporal order within auditory sequences. *Perception & Psychophysics*, 1972, **12**, 86-90.

Warren, R. M., Obusek, C. J., & Ackroff, J. M. Auditory induction: Perceptual synthesis of absent sounds. *Science*, 1972, **176**, 1149-1151.

Warren, R. M., Obusek, C.J., Farmer, R. M., & Warren, R.P. Auditory sequence: Confusion of patterns other than speech or music. *Science*, 1969, **164**, 586-587.

Warren, R. M., Sersen, E., & Pores, E. A basis for loudness-judgments. *American Journal of Psychology*, 1958, **71**, 700-709.

Warren, R. M., & Sherman, G. L. Phonemic restorations based on subsequent context. *Perception & Psychophysics*, 1974, **16**, 150-156.

Warren, R. M., & Warren, R. P. A comparison of speech perception in childhood, maturity, and old age by means of the verbal transformation effect. *Journal of Verbal Learning and Verbal Behavior*, 1966, **5**, 142-146.

Warren, R. M., & Warren, R. P. *Helmholtz on perception: Its physiology and development.* New York: Wiley, 1968.

Warren, R. M., & Warren, R. P. Auditory illusions and confusions. *Scientific American,* December 1970, **223,** 30-36.

Warren, R. M., & Wrightson, J. M. Stimuli producing conflicting temporal and spectral cues to frequency. *Journal of the Acoustical Society of America,* 1981, **70,** 1020-1024.

Wasserman, G. S. The physics of light and the physical correlate theory of sensory scaling. *Behavioral and Brain Sciences,* 1981, **4,** 210-211.

Watson, C. S. Factors in the discrimination of word-length auditory patterns. In S. K. Hirsh, D. H. Eldredge, and S. R. Silverman (Eds.), *Hearing and Davis: Essays honoring Hallowell Davis.* Saint Louis, Mo.: Washington University Press, 1976, 175-188.

Watson, C.S., Kelly, W. J., & Wroton, H. W. Factors in the discrimination of tonal patterns. II. Selective attention and learning under various levels of stimulus uncertainty. *Journal of the Acoustical Society of America,* 1976, **60,** 1176-1186.

Watson, C. S., Wroton, H. W., Kelly, W. J., & Benbassat, C. A. Factors in the discrimination of tonal patterns. I. Component frequency, temporal position, and silent intervals. *Journal of the Acoustical Society of America,* 1975, **57,** 1175-1185.

Wegel, R. L., & Lane, C. E. The auditory masking of one pure tone by another and its probable relation to the dynamics of the inner ear. *Physical Review,* 1924, **23,** 266-285.

Welford, A. T. *Ageing and human skill.* London: Oxford University Press, 1958.

Wever, E. G. *Theory of hearing.* New York: Wiley, 1949.

Wever, E. G., & Bray, C. Action currents in the auditory nerve in response to acoustical stimulation. *Proceedings of the National Academy of Sciences* (U.S.A.), 1930, **16,** 344-350.

Whitfield, I. C. Central nervous system processing in relation to spatio-temporal discrimination of auditory patterns. In R. Plomp and G. F. Smoorenburg (Eds.), *Frequency analysis and periodicity detection in hearing.* Leiden, The Netherlands: Sijthoff, 1970, 136-152.

Whitworth, R. H., & Jeffress, L.A. Time vs. intensity in the localization of tones. *Journal of the Acoustical Society of America,* 1961, **33,** 925-929.

Wickelgren, W. A. Context-sensitive coding, associative memory, and serial order in (speech) behavior. *Psychological Review,* 1969, **76,** 1-15.

Wiener, F. On the diffraction of a progressive wave by the human head. *Journal of the Acoustical Society of America,* 1947, **19,** 143-146.

Wier, C. C., & Green, D. M. Temporal acuity as a function of frequency difference. *Journal of the Acoustical Society of America,* 1975, **57,** 1512-1515.

Wightman, F. L. The pattern transformation model of pitch. *Journal of the Acoustical Society of America,* 1973, **54,** 407-416.

Wilcox, G. W., Neisser, U., & Roberts, J. Recognition of auditory temporal order. Paper presented at the Eastern Psychological Association, Boston, Spring 1972.

Wiley, R. L. *Speech communication using the strongly voiced components only.* Doctoral dissertation, Imperial College, University of London, 1968.

Willey, C. F., Inglis, E., & Pearce, C. H. Reversal of auditory localization. *Journal of Experimental Psychology,* 1937, **20,** 114-130.

Wilson, J. P., & Johnstone, J. R. Basilar membrane and middle-ear vibration in guinea pig measured by capacitive probe. *Journal of the Acoustical Society of America*, 1975, **57**, 705-723.

Winckel, F. *Music, sound and sensation: A modern exposition*. New York: Dover, 1967.

Wohlgemuth, A. On the after-effect of seen movement. *British Journal of Psychology, Monograph Supplement*. Cambridge, England: Cambridge University Press, 1911.

Woodworth, R. S. *Experimental Psychology*. New York: Holt, 1938.

Worchel, P., & Dallenbach, K. M. "Facial vision": Perception of obstacles by the deaf-blind. *American Journal of Psychology*, 1947, **60**, 502-553.

Worden, F. G. Hearing and the neural detection of acoustic patterns. *Behavioral Science*, 1971, **16**, 20-30.

Wright, D., Hebrank, J. H., & Wilson, B. Pinna reflections as cues for localization. *Journal of the Acoustical Society of America*, 1974, **56**, 957-962.

Wrightson, J. M., & Warren, R. M. Incomplete auditory induction of tones alternated with noise: Effects occurring below the pulsation threshold. *Journal of the Acoustical Society of America*, 1981, **69**, S105-S106 (Abstract).

Yost, W. A., & Hill, R. Strength of pitches associated with ripple noise. *Journal of the Acoustical Society of America*, 1978, **64**, 485-492.

Yost, W. A., Hill, R., & Perez-Falcon, T. Pitch and pitch discrimination of broadband signals with rippled power spectra. *Journal of the Acoustical Society of America*, 1978, **63**, 1166-1173.

Young, P. T. Auditory localization with acoustical transposition of the ears. *Journal of Experimental Psychology*, 1928, **11**, 399-429.

Yund, E. W., & Efron, R. Dichoptic and dichotic micropattern discrimination. *Perception & Psychophysics*, 1974, **15**, 383-390.

Zemlin, W. R. *Speech and hearing science: Anatomy and physiology*. (2nd Ed.) Englewood Cliffs, N.J.: Prentice-Hall, 1981.

Zurek, P. M. Spontaneous narrowband acoustic signals emitted by human ears. *Journal of the Acoustical Society of America*, 1981, **69**, 514-523.

Zwicker, E. Masking and psychological excitation as consequences of the ear's frequency analysis. In R. Plomp and G. F. Smoorenburg (Eds.), *Frequency analysis and periodicity detection in hearing*. Leiden, The Netherlands: Sijthoff, 1970, 376-396.

Zwislocki, J. J. Five decades of research on cochlear mechanics. *Journal of the Acoustical Society of America*, 1980, **67**, 1679-1685.

Zwislocki, J. J., & Kletsky, E. J. Tectorial membrane: A possible effect on frequency analysis in the cochlea. *Science*, 1979, **204**, 639-641.

Author Index

Subject Index

229

About the Author

The author received a Ph.D. in organic chemistry from New York University in 1951. After working on the chemical basis of taste for a few years, he decided that the behavior of organisms was more interesting than the behavior of molecules. During transitional years at Brown University (1954-1956) he had laboratories in the chemistry and the psychology departments. A Senior Postdoctoral Fellowship in physiological psychology, 1956-1958, marked his formal transformation from chemist to psychologist. His subsequent research in taste, vision, and hearing has been carried out at a number of institutions including: New York University College of Medicine; the Applied Psychology Unit of the Medical Research Council, Cambridge, England; Cambridge University; Oxford University; and the Psychology Laboratory of the National Institute of Mental Health, Bethesda, Maryland. He has formulated the physical correlate theory of sensory intensity, and has discovered a number of auditory phenomena including the phonemic restoration effect and the verbal transformation effect. His most recent research has dealt with mechanisms underlying the perception of acoustic sequences and their relation to speech perception, and also with the bases for perception of pitch and what he has called "infrapitch." He has published numerous articles and book chapters, and he and his wife, Roslyn Pauker Warren, are authors of the book, "Helmholtz on Perception: Its Physiology and Development" (Wiley, 1968). He has been at the University of Wisconsin-Milwaukee since 1964, and has been Distinguished Professor of Psychology since 1975.